Handbook of Nursing Research and Biostatistics

Handbook of Nursing Research and Biostatistics

Vaishali D Tendolkar

RN RM MSN (Psychiatric Nursing)

Lecturer
Department of Psychiatric Nursing
SRMM College of Nursing, Sawangi (Meghe)
Wardha, Maharashtra, India

JAYPEE BROTHERS MEDICAL PUBLISHERS

The Health Sciences Publisher

New Delhi | London

Jaypee Brothers Medical Publishers (P) Ltd

Headquarter
Jaypee Brothers Medical Publishers (P) Ltd
EMCA House, 23/23-B
Ansari Road, Daryaganj
New Delhi - 110 002, India
Landline: +91-11-23272143,+91-11-23272703,
+91-11-23282021,+91-11-23245672
Email: jaypee@jaypeebrothers.com

Corporate Office
Jaypee Brothers Medical Publishers (P) Ltd
4838/24, Ansari Road, Daryaganj
New Delhi 110 002, India
Phone: +91-11-43574357
Fax: +91-11-43574314
Email: jaypee@jaypeebrothers.com
Website: www.jaypeebrothers.com
Website: www.jaypeedigital.com

Overseas Office
J.P. Medical Ltd
83 Victoria Street, London
SW1H 0HW (UK)
Phone: +44 20 3170 8910
Fax: +44 (0)20 3008 6180
Email: info@jpmedpub.com

Inquiries for bulk sales may be solicited at: jaypee@jaypeebrothers.com

Handbook of Nursing Research and Biostatistics

First Edition: 2011, Reprint 2025

ISBN 978-93-5025-157-7

Printed in India

To

All the Budding Researchers

in Nursing

Foreword

With the persistent rise in evidence-based nursing practice, nursing research has gained momentum in all fields of nursing. Nurses, as practice nurses in the variety of clinical settings and also as educators in the classrooms, are becoming more and more research savvy. Gone are the days of accepting the rationales provided by seniors just by virtue of their authority. This is not the era of trial and error either. Today, in this space age, we as nurses must demand and strive for scientific solutions to the problems in the nursing field.

To achieve this status of methodical enquirer, nursing research is the need of time and hence, has become part of nursing curricula at diploma in nursing as well as at undergraduate and postgraduate levels.

Handbook of Nursing Research and Biostatistics by Vaishali D Tendolkar provides budding researchers of any curricula with learning material in nursing research in a very simple language. The relevant diagram, sketches and flow charts make the learning of nursing research easy. The content is organized logically and provides a concrete view of the nursing research progression. The content covers major portion of the syllabi for the subject by most of the universities.

The book will prove to be extremely useful for basic nursing, postbasic nursing and diploma nursing students in preparing for their examinations in the subject as well as for conducting their research projects. It is useful to postgraduate students as a ready reckoner for their research projects.

Sudha A Raddi
Principal
KLES College of Nursing
Belgaum, Karnataka, India

Preface

As I traverse my journey to postgraduate studies in nursing after a wide gap of fifteen years, I felt that the complexity of the books deter the students of my age from reading and understanding the contents. The lengthy compound rather complex sentences with jargon of word induced sleep at most attempts of study. The idea of a research book conceived in my mind during this period for the ones like me who, I supposed must be sailing in the same boat. My hobby of reading and attempting to cross the boundaries of dished out knowledge have helped me sail smoothly so far. It was always has been hard work and self-directed learning that provided challenge to my brain to attempt something different. The philosophy was to trade a new path rather than to be a follower at all times.

Being part of noble profession of nursing and encountered with the words *your presence should make a difference* that always triggered me for something different. This little venture is an outcome of those efforts.

I am sure that the simple language of the book which constitutes my notes on research and biostatistics would appeal to one and all; those who travel the research path and contribute to the nursing knowledge in their own ways.

The readers and researchers using the book are requested to contribute and correspond freely for the improvement of the book. Your valuable suggestions and guidance is required for the enhancement of our own professional community.

With regards and anticipation of encouragement from all.

Vaishali D Tendolkar

Acknowledgments

I would like to express my deep gratitude to M/s Jaypee Brothers Medical Publishers (P) Ltd. for bringing my long cherished dream into reality. I take this privilege to thank my teacher, Mrs Tapti Bhattacharjee (Retd. Major — MNS) Principal, Bharati Vidyapeeth's College of Nursing for being primary inspiration for the book.

I express my gratitude to my friend, Sudha Raddi, Principal, KLES College of Nursing, Belgaum, Karnataka, India for writing encouraging foreword to this first venture of mine.

I thank the management of Meghe Group for providing facilities and support, so that the book reaches its final shape.

My parents, mother-in-law, and other relatives have always been with me with their blessings showering on me.

A special word of thanks for my husband, Dinesh Tendolkar and my daughter, Nupoor, who have been a constant source of support all through the processing of the book.

Lastly, I express my gratitude to all my colleagues for providing timely peer review of the script of the book and their extensive help.

I remain indebted to God almighty for equipping me with strength and wisdom as I take this little step in my professional career.

Contents

CHAPTER 1

Introduction to Nursing Research

Nursing experiences a remarkable change in all parts of the world over the period of time. The demands on the nursing practice are ever increasing due to advancements in medical technology, the legal implications of nursing practice and cultural migration for variety of reasons. Nursing research has gained momentum in last few decades owing to these demands to meet the ever-changing demands of the nursing practice. Nursing research provides answers to these challenges in the most scientific manner.

RESEARCH

Research is defined as a systematic inquiry that uses disciplined methods to answer questions or solve problems.

GOALS OF RESEARCH

- To develop the body of knowledge.
- To refine the existing body of knowledge.
- To expand the body of knowledge in any given field.

RESEARCH TERMINOLOGY

Subjects: People being studies = study participants = respondents of questionnaire = sample = informants = key informants.

Researcher: Person who conducts the research— investigator

Collaborative research: Research conducted by a research team where the team consists of more than one researcher. The team members may be from the same field or from different disciplines.

Reviewer: An expert who critiques various aspects of a study and offers feedback.

Funder (sponsor): One who provides money/finances for conducting the research.

Naturalistic setting (in the field): Homes, places of work etc. These are locations of data collection from the subjects or areas of work at the time of data collection.

Laboratory setting: Highly controlled setting.

Site: Overall location for the research.

Abstractions: In quantitative research it means concepts and in qualitative research it means phenomenon.

Construct: Refers to an abstraction or mental representation inferred from situations or behaviors. Constructs are abstractions deliberately and systematically invented for specific purpose.

Theory: A theory is a systematic, abstract explanation of some aspects of reality. In a theory concepts are knitted together into a coherent system to describe or explain some aspects of the world.

Heterogeneous group: When an attribute is extremely varied in the group under study.

Homogeneous group: The amount of variability is limited in a group under study.

VARIABLES

Variable— Concepts are called variables in quantitative studies. A variable is something that varies.

Nearly all aspects of human being are variables. People and conditions vary and hence research is conducted. Researchers seek to understand how or why things vary and to learn how differences in one variable are related to differences in another. The degree of variability or heterogeneity of a group of subjects has implications for study design.

Variables are inherent characteristics of research subjects, e.g. age, blood group, weight, height, are attribute variables.

Many a times the researcher creates a variable.

TYPES OF VARIABLES

Continuous variable: Continuous variables have values along a continuum. It can assume an infinite number of values between two points, e.g. weight.

Discrete variable: It has finite number of values between any two points, representing discrete quantities, e.g. Number of children.

Categorical variables: These variables take on a small range of values that do not represent quantity, e.g. Blood Groups – 4 types.

Dichotomous variable: These are categorical variables that take on only two values, e.g. gender — male/female.

Dependent variable: It is the presumed effect. Also called outcome variable.

Independent variable— Presumed cause

- Variability in the dependent variable is presumed to depend on variability in the independent variable.
- Independent variable and dependent variable are the terms used to indicate direction of influence at times.
- Many dependent variables have multiple causes or antecedents.
- Variables are not inherently dependent or independent.
- A dependent variable in one study could be an independent variable in another.

CONCEPTUAL DEFINITION

A conceptual definition presents the abstract or theoretical meaning of the concepts being studied.

- In qualitative studies, conceptual definitions of key phenomena may be the major end product of the endeavor, reflecting an intent to have the meaning of concepts defined by those being studied.
- In quantitative studies, researchers must clarify and define concepts at the beginning.

OPERATIONAL DEFINITION

An operational definition of a concept specifies the operations that researchers must perform to collect and measure the required information.

- Operational definitions should be congruent with conceptual definitions, e.g. weight is defined as the amount that an object weighs in pounds measured to the nearest pound using a spring scale with subjects fully undressed after 10 hours of fasting.

- Definitional precision has the advantage of communicating exactly what terms mean within the context of the study.

DATA

Research data are the pieces of information obtained during a study.

The actual values of the study variables constitute the data.

Quantitative data: Information in numeric form.

Qualitative data: Narrative descriptions.

RELATIONSHIPS

Researchers explore or test relationships between the concepts.

A relationship is a bond or a connection between the concepts of the phenomena under study.

In Quantitative Studies

- Researchers are primarily interested in the relationship between the independent and dependent variables.
- Variation in the dependent variable is systematically related to variation in the independent variable and focused in the research question.
- Relationships are expressed in quantitative terms like less than, more than etc.
- Most of the quantitative studies are undertaken:
  - To determine whether relationships exist among variables.
  - To study the direction of the relationships.
  - To know the strength of the relationship.
  - To understand the nature of the relationship.
- Not all the relationships between variables can be interpreted as cause and effect relationships.
- There can be functional relationship or associative relationship between the variables.

In Qualitative Studies

- There is no quantifying of relationships, nor is there testing causal relationships.

- Researchers in qualitative studies seek patterns of association.
- Patterns of interconnected themes and processes are identified as a means of understanding the whole.

NURSING RESEARCH

Nursing research is defined as systematic inquiry designed to develop trustworthy evidence about issues of importance to the nursing profession, including nursing practice, education, administration and informatics.

IMPORTANCE OF RESEARCH IN NURSING

- There is broad support for evidence-based nursing practice.
- There is general understanding that research findings from rigorous studies provide strong evidence for informing nurse's decision and actions.
- Nursing actions and decisions based on evidence indicate that the actions are clinically appropriate, cost-effective and result in positive outcomes for clients.
- Nurses can provide very high quality nursing care and elevate the standard and reputation of the nursing profession with the help of nursing research findings.
- Integration of nursing research with evidence-based practice into the delivery of nursing care and the framework for nursing administration decision-making may help nursing achieve a 'Magnet' status.
- Changes to nursing practice are regularly occurring due to evidence-based practice.
- Clinical changes in large scale are occurring due to accumulation of research evidence about beneficial practice innovations.

SCOPE OF NURSING RESEARCH

The scope of nursing research may be studied as the consumer-producer continuum in nursing research. With current emphasis on EBP, every nurse must engage in one or more roles along a continuum of research participation.

Consumers of Nursing Research

At one end of this continuum are the nurses whose involvement in research is indirect. They are the users or consumers of nursing research. These consumers read research reports to develop new skills and to search for relevant findings that may affect their practice. This minimum involvement in nursing research must be maintained by all nurses.

EBP depends on well-informed nursing research consumers.

Producers of Nursing Research

At the other end of the continuum are the producers of the nursing research. These are nurses actively participating in designing and implementing studies in nursing practice, administration, and profession at large.

Earlier nursing educators were more involved in nursing research. Now a days research in nursing is increasingly conducted by practicing nurses who want to find out what works best for their patients.

Other Activities on the Continuum

A rich variety of research activities lie in between these two end points on the consumer–producer continuum (Fig. 1.1). The activities include:

- Participating in a journal club.
- Solving clinical problems and making clinical decisions based on rigorous research.
- Collaborating in the development of an idea for a clinical research project.
- Reviewing a proposed research plan.
- Offering clinical expertise to improve the research plan.
- Recruit the study participants.
- Assist in collecting research information.
- Guiding participants in studies.
- Discussing the implications and relevance of research findings with clients.

Nurses with some research skills are better than those without them, to make a contribution to nursing and to evidence-based practice. Understanding of nursing research can improve the depth and breadth of every nurse's professional practice.

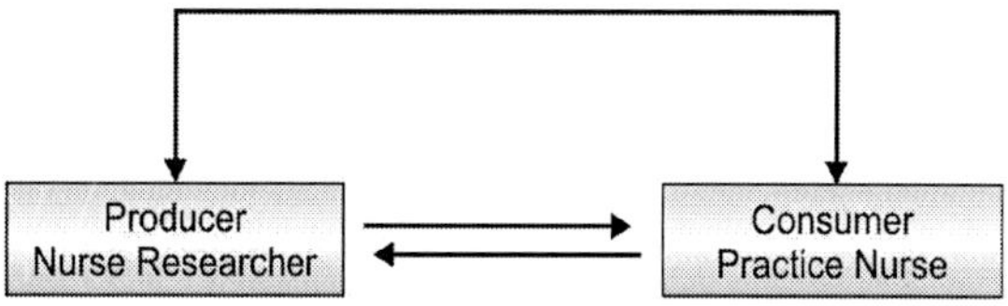

Fig 1.1 : Scope of nursing research continuum

HISTORICAL EVOLUTION OF RESEARCH IN NURSING

Research in nursing began with Florence Nightingale. Her 'Note on Nursing' in 1859 is the landmark publication. It describes environmental factors that promote physical and emotional wellbeing. She presented analysis of factors affecting soldier mortality and morbidity during Crimian war. Those were the findings that made her bring about changes in nursing care and public health.

Most of the studies in 1900s were concerned with nursing education. These identified many inadequacies in the educational background of the groups and concluded that advanced educational preparation was essential.

A number of forces combined during 1950s to put nursing research on a rapidly accelerating upswing in the United States. These included.

- Increase in the number of nurses with advanced educational degrees.
- Establishment of nursing research center at Walter Reed Army Institute of Research.
- Increase in the availability of funds for Nursing Research.
- The inception of American Nurses Foundation which is devoted exclusively to nursing research.
- The first journal "Nursing Research" published in 1952.

Nursing leaders began to express concern about the lack of research in nursing practice. Practice-oriented research on various clinical topics began to emerge in the literature. In the year 1963, International Journal of Nursing studies was published for the first time. By 1970, growing number of nurses conducting research studies created need for additional communication outlets. Hence, many research journals came into being.

During 1970s, a decided change in nursing research from areas of teaching, curriculum and nurses themselves to the improvement of client-care took place. This is considered as the modern foundation of scientific base for nursing practice.

By 1980, nursing research came to a new level of development. This decade is marked by:

- Increase in the qualified nurse researchers.
- Widespread availability of computers for the collection and analysis of information
- Ever-growing recognition of research being integral part of professional nursing.
- More attention to the types of questions, the methods of collecting and analyzing information being used, linking of research to theory and utilization of research findings in practice.
- The year 1986 is marked by establishment of National Center for Nursing Research in US.

NCNR–National Center for Nursing Research

The purpose of NCNR is to promote and financially support research projects and training relating to patient care. Clinical learning strategy called Evidence Based Practice was designed. EBP proved that research findings were far superior as a basis for clinical decisions and has had a significant effect on all health care professions including nursing.

Research specifically designed to improve the quality of health care, reduce health costs and enhance patient safety; were supported and promoted. In the year 1993, the NCNR became the National Institute of Nursing Research. This was important step towards strengthening the nursing research. Later in 1990s, there was emerging importance of in-depth studies using different methodologies. International cooperation about EBP in Nursing enhanced. The focus changed to research utilization.

FUTURE DIRECTIONS FOR NURSING RESEARCH

Nursing research continues to develop at a rapid pace. Funding for nursing research continues to grow. The priority for nursing research in the future will be the promotion of excellence in nursing science. Certain trends that have moulds been prepared are:

Heightened Focus on EBP

Efforts to use research findings in practice are sure to continue in coming era. Nurses are encouraged for EBP. Emerging interest is in translational research meaning research on how findings from studies can best be translated into nursing practice.

Development of a Stronger evidence-base through more Rigorous Methods and Multiple, Confirmatory Strategies

Strong research designs are essential for strong evidence. Confirmation of the evidence is required through replication of studies with different clients, in different clinical settings and at different times, to ensure that findings are robust. Multiple studies pose confirmatory strategy status.

Greater Emphasis on Systematic Integrative Review

Systematic reviews are cornerstone of EBP. Amassing comprehensive research information on the topic, weighing pieces of evidence and integrating information to draw conclusions about the state of evidence, is gaining importance in 21st century in the field of nursing practice.

Expanded Local Research in Health Care Setting

Increase in the small, localized research designed to solve immediate problems of the local clients. The local problems are influenced by a variety of factors including intrinsic, racial, social, cultural and constitutional in addition to external factors such as climate, geographical location etc. Mechanisms to ensure that evidence from these small projects, becomes available to others facing similar problems; need to be developed.

Strengthening of Multidisciplinary Collaboration

Interdisciplinary collaboration of nurses with researchers in related fields is must. Researchers address fundamental problems at the bio-behavioral and psychologic interface. Collaborative efforts could lead to nurse researcher playing a more prominent role in national and international health care policies.

Expanded Dissemination of Research Findings

The internet and other means of electronic communication have a large impact on the dissemination of research information, which in turn helps to promote EBP. Wide and quick access to the research information makes nurses well versed with the latest trends in nursing practice and the recent developments in the knowledge of nursing profession.

Increasing Visibility of Nursing Research

There are increased efforts to increase the visibility of nursing research. Most people do not know that nurses are scholars and researchers. Nurses must market their knowledge and their research to professional organizations in order to improve their social scholarly status.

Increasing Focus on Cultural Issues and Health Disparities

The issue of health disparities has emerged as a central concern in nursing and other health disciplines. This has raised consciousness about ecological validity and cultural sensitivity of health interventions.

Ecological validity refers to the extent to which study designs and findings have relevance and meaning in a variety of real world contexts.

Nursing research must be sensitive to the health beliefs, behaviors, epidemiology and values of culturally and linguistically diverse populations. Meeting the health care needs of an increasingly diverse society and a more globalized world has become an international concern.

PARADIGMS FOR NURSING RESEARCH

Paradigms	World view, General perspective
Ontologic	What is the nature of reality?
Epistemologic	What is the relationship between the inquirer and that being studied?
Axiologic	What is the role of values in the inquiry?
Methodologic	How should the inquirer obtain knowledge?

There are two paradigms for nursing research

1. Positivist
2. Naturalistic

Positivist Paradigm

- Dominated nursing research for decades.
- Also called logical positivism.
- Guided by philosophers like Comte, Newton, Mill and Locke.
- Scientific and modernism is the focus.

Definition: Positivism is a reflection of a broader cultural phenomenon that is referred to as modernism, which emphasizes the national and the scientific.

Major Concepts

- There exists reality.
- Reality in the world can be studied and known.
- Nature is basically ordered and regular.
- Objective reality exists independent of human observations.
- Phenomena have antecedent causes.
- Research is directed at understanding the underlying causes of natural phenomena.
- Positivists believe in objective reality and attempt to hold their personal belief and biases in check.
- Research involves the use of orderly, disciplined procedures with tight controls over the research situations.
- Study the nature of phenomena and the relationship among its concepts.
- Believe in reality and have a desire to understand it.
- Recognize the impossibility of total objectivity.

- But objectivity is their goal and they strive to be as neutral as possible.
- Appreciate the impediments to know reality.
- Hence also seek probabilistic evidence, i.e. probable true state of the phenomena under study.
- Quantitative research is most closely associated with positivism.

Definition: Scientific Method — Positivist scientific method refers to a general set of orderly, disciplined procedures used to acquire information.

- In a systematic study, the investigator progress logically through a series of steps, according to a pre-specified plan of action.
- Control involves imposing conditions on the research situation so that biases are minimized and precision and validity are maximized.
- Quantitative researcher gather empirical evidence, i.e. the evidence rooted in objective reality and gathered directly or indirectly through the senses – sight, hearing, taste, touch or smell.
- Information gathered is quantitative – numeric information that is analyzed with statistical procedures.
- The degree to which research findings can be generalized to individuals other than those who participated in the study (referred to as the generalizability of the research) is the criteria for assessing the quality of quantitative studies.
- Reflects the cultural phenomenon of modernism in the wake of the industrial revolution.
- It is a reductionist model as it reduces human experiences to only the few concepts under investigation.

The Naturalistic Paradigm

- Also called constructivist paradigm
- Promoted by writers – Weber and Kant

Definition: Naturalism is an outgrowth of the pervasive cultural transformation called postmodernism.

- Emphasizes deconstruction — taking apart old ideas and structures and reconstruction — putting ideas and structures together in new ways.

- Reality is not a fixed entity.
- Reality exists within a context and many constructions are possible.
- There are multiple interpretations of reality.
- There is no process by which the ultimate truth or falsity of the construction can be determined.
- Knowledge is maximized when the distance between the inquirer and the participants in the study is minimized.
- Voices and interpretations of those under study are crucial to understanding the phenomenon of interest.
- The findings are the products or interactions between the inquirer and the participants. The naturalistic methods deal with the human complexity by exploring it directly. The truth is composite of realities.
- It believes in and attempts to understand the human experience as it is lived.
- Careful collection and analysis of qualitative materials that are narrative and subjective is must.
- Naturalistic researchers emphasize the dynamic, holistic and individual aspects of human experiences.
- They capture the entire experience within the context of those who are experiencing them.
- Flexible, evolving procedures and findings that emerge in the course of investigations.
- Inquiry takes place in the field over an extended period of time.
- Collection of information and its analysis typically progress concurrently.
- Through inductive process, researchers integrate information to develop a theory or description that helps to explain the phenomena under observation.
- Studies yield rich, in-depth information.
- Findings are grounded in the real-life experiences of people with first hand knowledge of the phenomenon.
- Human beings are used directly as the instrument.
- Subjective nature of naturalistic inquiry.
- Idiosyncratic nature of conclusions.
- Relatively small group of people under study.
- Generalizability of findings may be limited.

IMPORTANT POINTS TO BE NOTED

Both, qualitative and quantitative research methods cannot be used to answer moral or ethical questions, e.g. Euthanasia to be practiced or not.

Since many moral issues are linked to health care, it is inevitable that nursing process cannot rely exclusively on scientific information.

Accurate measures of psychological phenomena like hope, self-esteem are not yet developed.

Human beings are inherently complex and diverse, extremely intelligent, sensitive but fallible tools.

Quantitative research is accused of narrowness and inflexibility of vision, i.e. a sedimented view of the world that does not fully capture the reality of human experience.

GLOBAL NURSING PRIORITIES

Nursing is an important pillar of health care delivery system in all parts of the world. With the changing medical technology, the priorities in the nursing practice also change. The change in the nursing practice is so great that it influences the actual health care delivery by all the health team members. Some of the global nursing priorities are:

- Health promotion and disease prevention through health education and health awareness of masses.
- Promotion of health of vulnerable and marginalized communities.
- Patient safety and quality of health care.
- Development of EBP and translational research.
- Promotion of the health and well-being of older people.
- Patient centered care and care coordination.
- Palliative and end of life care.
- Care implications of genetic testing and genetic therapeutics.
- Capacity development of nurse researchers.
- Nurses' working environment.

PURPOSES OF NURSING RESEARCH

General purpose of nursing research is to answer the questions or solve problems of relevance to the nursing profession.

Specific purposes: Specific purposes of nursing research include:

- Basic research to extend the base of knowledge in nursing.
- To formulate or refine a nursing theory.
- Applied research to find solutions to existing problems.
- To enhance the immediate utility of EBP.
- To study the effectiveness of a nursing interventions.
- To discover general principles of human behavior to solve problems in nursing practice.
- To achieve varying levels of explanation.
- To identify, describe, explore, explain and predict and to exert control over the existing health problem situation.
- To link research findings with EBP.
- To develop and rigorously test a new method of measuring patient outcomes.
- To help nurses make evidence-based treatment decisions.
- To determine the benefits and risks of the newly developed or existing interventions.
- To assess the cost-effectiveness of nursing interventions
- To diagnose, assess patients and to measure important clinical outcomes.
- To facilitate the development of long-term care plans for patients.
- To provide guidance to patients to make important lifestyle choices and to be vigilant for key symptoms.
- To decide resource allocation.
- To prevent harm to the patients.
- To determine the factors that, influence the health or cause illness, mortality, morbidity.
- To design effective interventions.
- To motivate people to comply with the treatment.
- To engage in health promotion activities.
- To study the barriers to positive health practices.
- To understand the processes clients experience in a transition through health care crisis.

The purpose of research can be further studied depending on the nature of the study, i.e. the quantitative study or qualitative study.

PURPOSES OF QUANTITATIVE RESEARCH

- To assess the prevalence of phenomenon. (How much?)
- To study the frequency of the phenomenon. (How often?)
- To understand the nature of phenomenon. (What is?)
- To study the factors related to the phenomenon. (What influences?)
- To know the antecedents of the phenomenon. (What leads to?)
- To identify the causal pathway of the phenomenon.
- To apply theory to explain the phenomenon.
- To understand the alterations in the phenomenon with modification or introduction of an intervention.
- To predict the occurrence of cause and effect.
- To make the phenomenon occur or to alter its prevalence.

PURPOSES OF QUALITATIVE RESEARCH

- To define the phenomenon.
- To label the phenomenon.
- To understand the dimensions of the phenomenon.
- To know the important aspects of the phenomenon.
- To understand the nature of the phenomenon in depth.
- To study the events/outcomes to which the phenomenon leads.
- To illustrate the process by which the phenomenon evolves or is experienced.
- To identify what makes the phenomenon occur/exist.
- To study the working of the phenomenon.
- To learn the meaning of the phenomenon.
- To evaluate the occurrence of the phenomenon.

The nursing research, though a recently developed dimension of nursing profession; had existed ever since the nursing existed. From its most primitive trial and error form, it has evolved to today's most modern and scientific study. It is only three decades back it got momentum with the rapid inventions and technological advances in the health care delivery. From the transition of family doctor to family nurse, research literacy is vital for nurses to provide cost-effective managed care.

CHAPTER 2

Evidence-based Practice

For years the nursing students are guided for trial and found true basis in finding solutions to problems that are confronted for the first time in nursing practice. This is one of the most unscientific methods of nursing practice as people vary in their constitution and response to diseases in addition to the difference in clinical presentation of problem. People with different diseases may present with similar problems and clinical picture of same disease may vary in different people. This is where the nurse must have a strong evidence to practice an intervention safely for the client in order to enhance the progress towards recovery. Evidence-based practice (EBP) plays a vital role in this modern era of managed care where people are aware of their health problems and the available treatment modalities for their problems. People also have started making health decisions related to choosing a particular treatment modality without much alteration in the daily routine.

SOURCES OF EVIDENCE FOR NURSING PRACTICE

Nurses make clinical decisions based on knowledge and information. Faculty and textbooks are source of knowledge and information for nurses for their practice. Nurses learn from each other and from interactions with other health care professionals. Some of their learning is based on systematic research. About 85 percent of the health care practice is not validated and hence the need for evidence from research for practice is markedly felt. Information sources for clinical practice vary in dependability and validity. Evidence hierarchies (Fig. 2.1) are acknowledgement of certain types of evidence and knowledge superior to others.

Accordingly, following are the sources of evidence for nursing practice:

Tradition and Authority

In this, the decisions are made based on the customs or tradition. Each culture has certain 'truths' that are accepted as given. This facilitated communication by providing a common foundation of accepted truth. Many nursing interventions are based on tradition, customs and 'unit culture' rather than on sound evidence.

Another source of information is an authority where a person with specialized expertise and recognition for that expertise passes on the knowledge to those who approach and contact him/her to acquire the knowledge and expertise. Authorities are not infallible, but like tradition their knowledge goes unchallenged.

Clinical Experience

It is a familiar and functional source of knowledge. The ability to generalize, to recognize regularities and make predictions based on observation is common in clinical practice. Each nurse's experience is too narrow to be generally useful. Nurses may have different opinions and views of the same event. In addition, people have individual differences in response to health and illness.

Trial and Error

Alternatives are tried successfully until a solution to a problem is found. It offers a practical means of securing knowledge; but is fallible. It is a haphazard method and the solutions may be idiosyncratic. Evidences are usually unrecorded and hence inaccessible in subsequent clinical situations.

Intuition

Intuition is a type of knowledge that cannot be explained on the basis of reasoning or prior instruction. It is difficult to develop policies and practices for nurses on the basis of intuition.

Logical Reasoning

Solutions of many problems are found by logical thought processes. It combines experience, intellectual faculties and formal systems of thought.

Two types of logical reasoning are practiced by the nurses while making clinical decisions. They are inductive reasoning and deductive reasoning.

Inductive reasoning: It is a process of developing generalizations from specific observations, e.g. anxious behavior of hospitalized children is observed and concluded that children's separation from their parents is stressful.

Deductive reasoning: It is the process of developing specific predictions from general principles, e.g. if it is assumed that hospitalized children experience anxiety of separation from their parents in general then in a specific hospital, the hospitalized children would also show signs of anxiety and stress due to hospitalization and separation from their parents.

Both the systems of reasoning are useful to understand and organize a phenomenon. Both play active role in nursing research and nursing practice. Validity of reasoning depends on the accuracy of the information.

Assembled Information

Clinical decisions are guided by the information assembled for a variety of purposes, e.g. local, national and international bench-marking data provide information about morbidity and mortality rates, etc. and serve as a guide in evaluating clinical practices.

Cost data are sometimes used for clinical decision making. Quality improvement and risk data can be used to assess practices and determine the need for practice changes.

Disciplined Research

Research conducted within a disciplined format is the most sophisticated method of acquiring knowledge. Nursing research combines aspects of logical reasoning with other features to create evidence. In this case the evidence is more reliable. Cumulative findings from rigorous and systematically appraised research are at the pinnacle of most evidence hierarchies. Nursing will always remain a rich blend of art and science.

EVIDENCE-BASED PRACTICE (EBP)

Evidence-based practice is the conscientious use of current best evidence in making clinical decision about patient care. It is synonymous with translating research evidence into nursing practice.

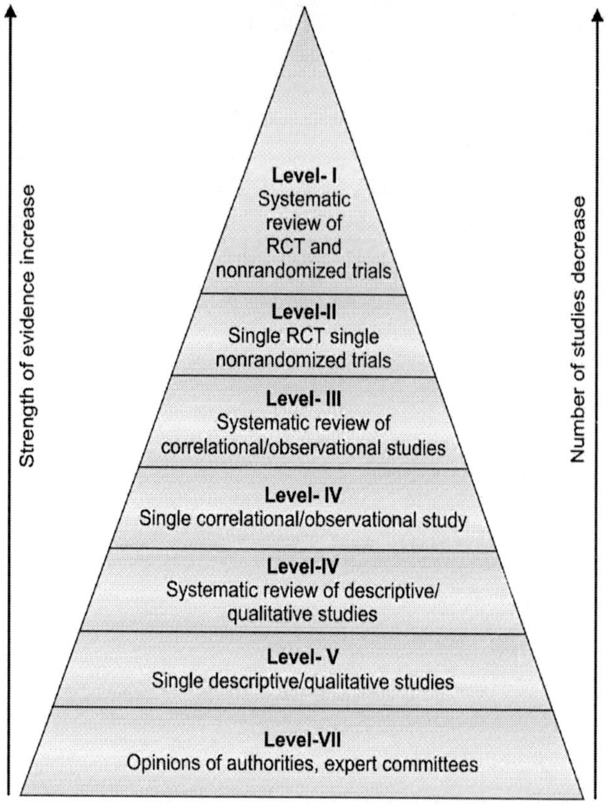

Fig 2.1 : Evidence hierarchy

NATURE OF EBP

Research evidence provides invaluable insights about human health and illness. Nurses and other health care professionals must be lifelong learners of the skill to search for, understand and evaluate new information about patient care. Nurse must have capacity to be flexible and to adapt to changes. EBP de-emphasizes decisions based on customs, authority, opinion or ritual.

EBP emphasizes on identifying the best available research evidence and integrating it with other factors. EBP does not minimize the importance of clinical expertise. Evidence-based decision making integrates best research evidence with clinical expertise, patient preferences and circumstances and awareness of the clinical setting and resource constraints. EBP is the effort to personalize the evidence to fit a specific patient's needs and a particular clinical situation. EBP starts with a clinical question and results in finding a number of solutions to it.

RESEARCH UTILIZATION

Research utilization is the use of findings from a disciplined study or set of studies in a practical application that is unrelated to the original research. Research utilization emphasizes on translating empirically derived knowledge into real-world applications. Research utilization begins with the research.

It is a systematic process used by nurses to incorporate research based knowledge into professional nursing practice.

Need for Research Utilization

- New knowledge is generated rapidly.
- Learnt material during educational program may become obsolete within few years.
- Professional nurses cannot plead ignorance of new knowledge and practices.
- Nurses are accountable to their profession and need to update their knowledge to practice appropriately.

Advantages of Research Utilization

- A sound foundation for practice.
- Enhanced self-confidence, autonomy, critical thinking skills and professional self-concept.
- Cost–effective patient care.
- Increased patient and job satisfaction and quality of care.
- Improved patient outcomes.
- A stimulus for collaborative practice, retention and recruitment.
- An improved image of nursing.
- An ever increasing scientific nursing knowledge base.

Types of Research Utilization

a. **Indirect research utilization—** It involves changes in nurse's thinking.
b. **Direct research utilization—** It involves the direct use of research findings in giving patient care.
c. **Persuasive research utilization—** It involves the use of findings to persuade others to make changes in policies or practices relevant to nursing care.

EBP IN NURSING

EBP offers solution to improving health care quality in our current cost-constrained environment. A rationale approach is needed to provide the best possible care to the most people, with the most cost-effective use of resources. EBP provides an important framework for self-directed lifelong learning that is need of the time with rapid clinical advances and the information explosion.

In the EBP environment, a skillful clinician can no longer rely on a repository of memorized information, but must gain skills in accessing, evaluating, synthesizing and using new research evidence. Findings from rigorous research are of paramount importance. Evidence hierarchies rank evidence sources according to the strength of the evidence they provide. The strongest evidence according to evidence hierarchy comes from systematic reviews that integrate findings from multiple studies using rigorous and methodological procedures.

Systematic reviews of nonrandomized clinical trials offer less powerful evidence. The evidence hierarchy is appropriate with regard to questions about the effects of clinical interventions or treatments. In nursing, the best evidence refers to findings from research that are methodologically appropriate, rigorous and clinically relevant for answering questions. The questions are not only about the efficacy, safety and cost-effectiveness of nursing interventions, but also about the reliability of nursing assessment measures, the determinants of health and wellbeing, the meaning of health or illness and the nature of patient's experience.

Confidence in the evidence is enhanced when the research methods are compelling, with multiple confirmatory replication studies and when the evidence is systematically evaluated and synthesized. When sufficient research information is not available for a certain nursing question, then nursing practice must rely on other sources like bench-marking data, chart review, clinical expertise, etc. One benefit of EBP is that, when a clinical question with no satisfactory evidence, arise, a new research agenda can result.

RESOURCES FOR EBP

There are various resources for the evidence based practice in nursing. Some of them are as follows:

Systematic Reviews

EBP relies on meticulous integration of research evidence on a topic. The emphasis on best evidence in EBP implies that all evidence about a clinical problem has been gathered, evaluated and synthesized so that conclusions can be drawn about effective practices.

A systematic review is in itself a methodical, scholarly inquiry that follows the steps involved in primary study. Systematic reviews on a wide variety of clinical topics are increasingly available and represent a rich resource for EBP. Evidence reports to help improve the quality, effectiveness and appropriateness of clinical care.

The most common type of systematic review was traditional narrative (qualitative) integration to merge and synthesize research findings. These are of two types namely – Meta-analysis and Meta-synthesis.

Meta-analysis: It is the technique for integrating quantitative research findings statistically. Meta-analysis treats the findings from a study as one piece of information. The findings from multiple studies on the same topic are combined, and the obtained information is analyzed statistically in the manner similar to that in a routine study. Thus, the individual studies are the units of analysis in a meta-analysis. It provides a convenient and objective method of integrating a large body of findings and of observing patterns that might otherwise have gone undetected. It is more of reducing information.

Meta-synthesis: A meta-synthesis involves integrating qualitative research findings on a specific topic that are themselves interpretive syntheses of narrative information. It is more about amplifying and interpreting information.

Clinical Practice Guidelines

Evidence-based clinical practice guidelines represent a large body of evidence into a manageable form. Clinical practice guidelines give specific practice recommendations and prescriptions for evidence-based decision making. Primarily, they influence clinician's activities. Secondly, they attempt to address all the issues relevant to a clinical decision, including the balancing of benefits and risks. Thirdly, they are necessity driven, meaning they are developed to guide practice.

Guidelines define a minimum set of services and actions appropriate for certain clinical conditions. Guidelines allow a flexible approach in their application to patients. To find, appraise and implement a clinical practice guideline involves a lot of work and collaboration. Guidelines-driven care in nursing is effective in improving some processes and outcomes of care. Multiple guidelines on the same topic are available for clinicians to choose from. Different guidelines may offer different and even conflicting recommendations. Hence, clinical practice guidelines must be critically appraised to identify ones with strongest evidence, meticulously developed, user friendly and appropriate for local use or adaptation.

Other Pre-appraised Evidence

These include:

1. Synopsis of systematic reviews
2. Synopses of single studies
3. Critical Summaries of studies and systematic reviews
4. Evidence-based medical reviews
5. Evidence digest, etc.

RESEARCH FINDINGS ON EBP

Research about EBP and the process of translating research into practice is a rich resource in planning an EBP. This body of research has been diverse, including both qualitative and quantitative studies. The studies related to factors that are barriers or facilitators of EBP have been widely conducted. Findings of these studies suggest the areas that can aid in the promotion of EBP. Nurses must be aware of the issues that need to be addressed in advancing evidence based nursing practice.

FACTORS INFLUENCING RESEARCH UTILIZATION

- Beliefs and attitudes towards nursing research.
- Involvement in nursing research activities.
- Information seeking behavior.
- Education level.
- Professional characteristics.
- Socioeconomic factors.
- Organizational factors

Organizational Factors

- Clear expectation of RU as a part of job description
- Staff educational programs on the process of research utilization.
- Incentives, such as promotions or salary increases.
- Formation of RU committees.
- Provision of time for nurses to read research reports while on duty.
- Clinical career ladders requiring RU as criteria for promotion and maintenance of organizational position.
- Organizational support to defray expenses for RU projects.
- Formalized collaboration between nursing service and academics.
- Library services for nurses to use to perform computerized literature searches and access needed materials.
- Nursing unit based libraries and nursing journal subscriptions.
- Sponsorship of nurses to attend professional nursing conferences.

BARRIERS TO RESEARCH UTILIZATION

RU barriers are any factors that block or impede the use of research findings in clinical practice. Following factors are major barriers.

Nature of Disseminated Research Studies

- Insufficient current research for today's complex clinical problems.
- Failures of replica research studies.
- Difficult research reports.

- Unpublished or non disseminated research reports.
- Lack of central depository for nursing research studies.

Characteristics of the Clinician

- Lack of education in how to read, critique, conduct and use research.
- Negative attitudes among practicing nurses.
- Not enough time or commitment to implement research utilization projects.
- Failure of nurses to read nursing research articles or journals.
- Inability of nurses to understand statistical analysis contained within studies.
- Comfort with practice based on tradition (even if ineffective).
- Difficulty, determining if studies are well designed and scientifically sound.
- Isolation from knowledgeable colleagues who could assist them in understanding research studies.
- Failure to understand statistics.

Nurse Researcher Characteristics

- Submission of studies for publication to journals not read widely by most nurses.
- Failure to offer realistic implications for clinical practice.
- Presentation of findings in a format not conducive to clinical implementation.

The Health Care Agency Administration

- Minimal value placed on research by many administrators.
- No provision for resources such as time, financial support and education.
- Lack of nursing autonomy.
- Lack of incentives.
- Reliance on established policy and procedures.
- Lack of support for implementation of research findings by physicians and other staff.

Some other barriers to utilization of research findings are enlisted below:

- High quality research evidence is limited.

- Researches with issues of generalizability are many.
- There are issues of limited or inadequate collaboration between researchers and clinicians.
- Nurse researchers need to improve their ability to communicate their findings.
- Nurses attitudes and education is a consistent potential barrier.
- Nurses do not value research or believe in the benefits of EBP.
- Nurses are resistant to change their practices.
- Many nurses do not know how to access research information while others do not possess the skills to critically evaluate research findings.
- Nurses do not know to effectively incorporate research evidence into clinical decision making.
- Lack of English-language skills is also a barrier as most of the research evidence is reported in English.
- Many of the impediments to use research in practice are organizational.
- Many organizations support the idea of EBP in theory, but may not provide the necessary support in terms of staff release time and resources.
- Commitment on the part of the managers and administrators is a must to make EBP a part of organizational norms.
- Strong leadership in health care organizations is essential to make EBP happen.

RESEARCH CRITIQUE

A research critique is a careful appraisal of the strengths and weaknesses of a study. A good critique objectively identifies areas of adequacy and inadequacy, virtues as well as faults of a study.

Purposes of Research Critique

- To record factual information about studies, their methodologic features and findings.
- To make judgements about the worth of the studies evidence.
- For students to critique a study as a part of their curriculum.
- To provide an evidence of student's/critique's mastery of methodologic concepts.

- To cultivate critical thinking.
- To induce students to use newly acquired skills in research methods.
- To obtain documentation of students skills in research methods.
- To prepare students for a professional nursing career.
- To gain skills in evaluating the research proposals of students.
- To develop an EBP.
- To evaluate the integrity of a study's evidence.
- To formulate the base for newer study.

Dimensions of Research Critique

Research problem: Whether the problem has significance for nursing.

- Whether the problem has the potential to produce evidence to improve nursing practice.
- Whether the research problem is compatible with the chosen research paradigm and its associated methods.
- Whether the research question and statement of purpose worded properly.
- Whether the hypotheses are logically connected to the research problem.
- Whether hypotheses are consistent with available knowledge or relevant theory.

Broad Dimensions of Research Critique

- Substantive and theoretical aspects
- Ethical issues
- Methodologic decisions
- Interpretation
- The report's organization, thoroughness and presentation.

Substantive and theoretical aspects: Substantive aspects include pattern, qsuantity, consistency, power, persuasiveness and gaps in the body of evidence.

Theoretical aspects include: Theoretical framework used and interrelationship of constructs are congruent with theoretical framework.

Findings vary in relation to difference in:

Theoretical Framework

At times the study may be atheoretical, i.e. no theoretical framework used to explain the interrelation between constructs (This followed by ethical issues).

Ethical Issues

- Research done with adequate authentic permissions.
- Research passed by Institutional Ethical Board.
- Suggestions by the Institutional Ethical Board implemented.
- Informed consent taken.
- Rights of the subjects catered to.
- Confidentiality ensured.

Methodologic Decisions

- Design of study and method used.
- Methodologic deficiencies and strengths.
- Methodologic features used to enhance the rigor.
- Commonalities and differences in methodologic features of rigorous studies.

Interpretation— It includes:

- Generalizability/transferability.
- Substantive, theoretical or methodologic trends over time.
- Time period of the research.
- Researcher's discipline, specialty area, nationality, prominence, etc.
- Development of research within a systematic program of research.

Organization and Presentation

- Presentation is logical.
- Demonstrates meaningful thematic integration.
- Leads to a conclusion.

OVERALL CRITIQUE OF RESEARCH

Quantitative Research Report

Title	Should be good, suggest key variables, suggest the study population.

Abstract	Clearly and concisely summarize the main features—problem, method, results, conclusions.
Introduction	Statement of problem, hypotheses of research question, literature review, conceptual / theoretical framework.
Method	Protection of participant's rights, research design, population and sample, data collection and measurement, procedures.
Results	Data analysis, findings.
Discussion	Interpretations of the findings, implications and recommendations.
Global issues	Presentation, researcher credibility, summary assessment.

Overall strengths and weaknesses of the study should be commented.

Qualitative Research Report

Title	Should be good, suggest key phenomenon, Group or community under study.
Abstract	Clearly and concisely summarize the main features.
Introduction	Statement of the problem, research question, Literature review, conceptual underpinning.
Method	Ethical issues, research design and tradition, Sample and setting, data collection, procedures — minimal bias for data collection, enhancement of rigor–trustworthiness.
Results	Data analysis—theory, taxonomy, thematic pattern, etc. possibility of biases, finding, theoretical integration,
Discussion	Interpretations of the findings, implications and recommendations.
Global issues	Presentation, researcher credibility, summary assessment.

EBP IN INDIVIDUAL NURSING PRACTICE

Individual nurses make many decisions, provide health care advice and thus have ample opportunity to put research into practice, to improve the quality of nursing care.

For individual level EBP efforts, the major steps in EBP include–

- Asking clinical questions that are answerable with research evidence.
- Searching for and collecting relevant evidence.
- Appraising and synthesizing the evidence.
- Integrating the evidence with your own clinical expertise, patient preferences and local context.
- Assessing the effectiveness of the decision, intervention or advice.

In India nursing practice is not empowered by knowledge. Traditional ways of practice are most common. This is because ANM and GNM trained staff nurses are in the clinical setting and knowledge professionals are in the classroom teaching. The fact is that in India there is wide scope for nursing research and evidence-based practice because of its varied cultural heritage. Refining the nursing knowledge is must with changes in the society and social needs. One must be ready to match with the present demands on health sector.

CHAPTER 3 Theoretical Bases for Nursing Research

Nursing theories have developed in last three decades as the awareness of nursing knowledge development grew. With the fast changing medical technology and the decentralization of health care delivery in the community, it became mandatory to expand discipline of nursing knowledge in diverse field. Today, nurses face a variety of clients and diseases they suffer which were not known in the past. Human quest for more productive longer life is growing everyday which has stimulated research for making life comfortable and more productive. Medical field is no exception and naturally nursing field cannot be an exception. This has resulted in finding theoretical bases for nursing research to improve, expand, refine existing nursing knowledge and to create new knowledge so that nurses provide evidence-based nursing care that matches quality.

THEORY

Theory is a creative and rigorous structuring of ideas that projects a tentative, purposeful and systematic view of phenomena.

IMPORTANCE OF NURSING THEORIES

Professional nurses apply concepts, principles and theories from many disciplines. Theories create a different way of looking at a particular phenomenon by interrating concepts in a logical manner and provide a framework for describing, explaining and predicting practice.

Theories provide a simple and generalizable view for testable hypothesis development.

Validated theories expand discipline specific knowledge.

Theories aid to identify questions for future investigation.

They help to derive a rationale for nursing actions.

Theories provide a knowledge base for the science of nursing.

They aid to understand, explain, predict and control events related to health.

Application of a theory fosters the recognition of nursing as a professional discipline.

Model: The world view of change reflected by the model – Growth or stability.

Theory: The major theoretical/conceptual classification with which the model seems more consistent.

Some recognize change as continuous, a desired opportunity for growth to attain maximum human potential.

Others believe it to be persistence which maintains that persons strive for stability and that endurance results from a synthesis of growth and stability.

THE STABILITY MODEL OF CHANGE

Change is inevitable, it forces for adaptation.

The natural order of things revolves around consistency

Stability means that the organism attains a new and stable equilibrium.

GENERAL SYSTEMS THEORY

General systems theory is concerned with elements and interactions among all the factors (variables) in a situation.

It provides a way to understand the many influences on the whole person and the possible impact of change on any part of the whole.

Help nurses to understand, predict and control the possible effects of nursing care on the client system and the concurrent effects of the interaction on the nurse system and environment.

"A system is defined as a whole with interrelated parts, in which each part has some functions and the system as totality has function(s)."

Subsystem may be smaller than the tiniest cell of an organism.

Suprasystem extends beyond what human know as the universe.

The whole person is a suprasystem for multiple interacting subsystems (Bodily boundaries).

The person holds membership in a subsystem called family which is a subsystem of community system.

A subsystem may be isolated for study by human beings. It may be more than and different from the sum of its parts.

As open systems, persons exchange matter, energy and information across their boundaries with the environments.

A person's internal environment interacts constantly with an ever-changing external environment.

Changes in one affect the other.

Openness of human systems makes nursing interventions possible.

Constancy does not mean that the internal environment is static, but rather constantly changing.

The system seeks equilibrium or a steadystate, in which a balance exists among the various forces operating within and on the system (Fig. 3.1).

Factors from the environment impinge on the system across the system boundary resulting in tension, stress, strain or conflict that may upset system balance (Fig. 3.2).

Imogene King's Model/Theory of Goal Attainment

- Imogene King stresses interactions and mutuality in her nursing model.
- Developed when she was trying to outline essential content for a new graduate nursing program.

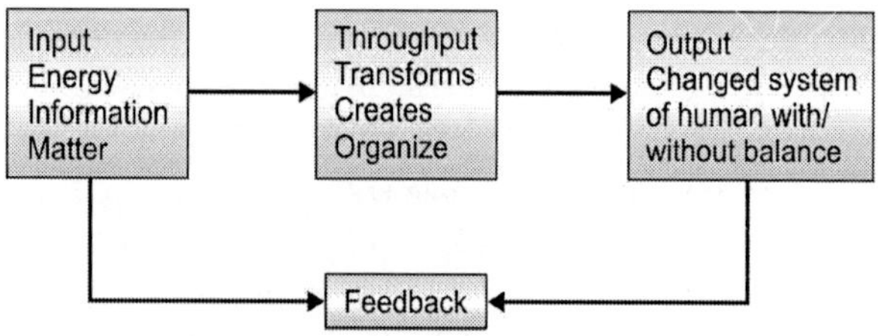

Fig. 3.1: General systems theory

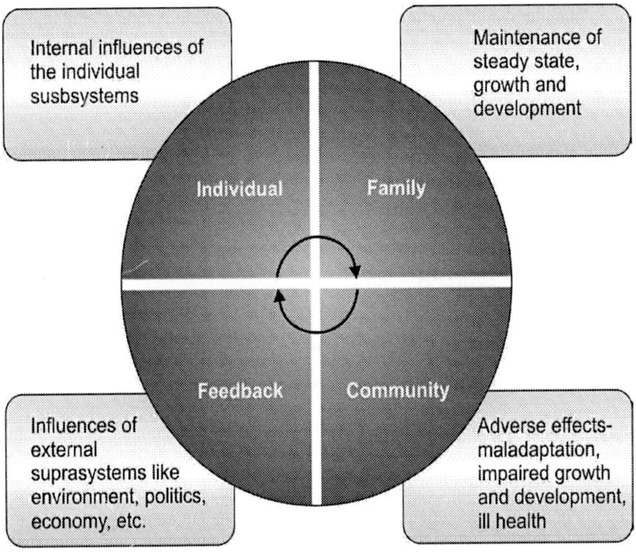

Fig. 3.2: Application of general systems theory

Purpose of Nursing

- To help people attain, maintain or restore health, primarily by mutual goal setting.
- Nurse-patient interaction is a transaction which includes nurse-patient mutual understanding of events, mutually set goals and agreement on means to achieve the goals.
- Roots in sociology.
- Focuses on individuals whose interactions in groups within social systems influence behavior within the system.
- Humans are defined as open systems interacting with environment.
- Human is rational, sentient, reacting, social, controlling, purposeful, time-oriented and action-oriented system.
- World is the total person = suprasystem resulting in environmental interactions to which he/she must constantly adjust.
- Environment is both internal as well as external.
- Each person is a whole system who interacts with one or more persons thereby creating internal system.

- Social systems are developed as interpersonal systems extend to include large groups of persons.
- The social system, the interpersonal systems and the person systems constantly interact with one another.
- Nurses interact with clients to facilitate achievement of mutually determined health related goals.
- Perception is comprehensive concept in personal systems.
- Interaction provides a channel for passage of information from one person to another.
- Concepts of self, growth and development, learning, body image, time and space relate to individual as personal systems.
- Interaction is the comprehensive concept in interpersonal systems.
- Dynamic life experiences of a human being which calls for continuous adjustment to stressors in the internal and external environment through optimum use of resources to achieve maximum potential for daily living.
- Illness causes imbalance in person's biological structure, psychological make up or a conflict in a person's social relationships.
- The goal of nursing is to help individuals and groups attain, maintain and restore health.
- Nursing care is rendered within goal-oriented nurse-patient interactions wherein actions indicate movement toward goal achievement.

Major Concepts in King's Model

- **Person (human being):** A personal system that interacts with interpersonal and social systems.
- **Environment:** A context within which human beings grow, develop and perform daily activities.
- **Health:** Dynamic life experiences of a human being, which implies continuous adjustment to stressors in the internal and external environment through optimum use of one's resources to achieve maximum potential for daily living.
- **Nursing:** A process of human interaction.

Ten Key Concepts of King's Theory

1. **Interaction:** A process of perception and communication between person and environment and between person and person, represented by verbal and nonverbal behaviors that are goal-oriented.
2. **Perception:** Each person's representation of reality.
3. **Communication:** A process whereby information is given from one person to another.
4. **Transaction:** An observable behavior of human beings interacting with their environment valuation is a component of human interaction.
5. **Role:** A sent of behaviors expected of persons occupying a position in a social system.
6. **Stress:** A dynamic state whereby a human being interacts with the environment to maintain balance for growth, development and performance.
7. **Growth and development:** Continuous change in individuals at the cellular, molecular and behavioral levels of activities.
8. **Time:** A continuous flow of events in successive order that implies change, a past and a future.
9. **Self:** A personal system defined as a unified complex whole.
10. **Space:** Existing in all directions and the same everywhere.

Mutual goal setting is a critical independent variable and goal attainment is the dependent one. The theory defines the process of mutual goal setting and strengths of mutual goal setting. It provides a theoretical base for application of traditional nursing process. It is used as a basis for many research projects in nursing performed internationally in the areas of decision-making processes for clients and effectiveness of client education. It provides foundation for UG, PG nursing programs and nursing service departments (Fig. 3.3).

BETTY NEWMAN'S HEALTH CARE SYSTEMS MODEL

Betty Newman developed her model while she attempted to help nursing students organize their thinking and look at clients holistically.

- The model specifies that the purpose of nursing is to facilitate optimal client system stability by reducing the impact of environmental stimuli or stressors.

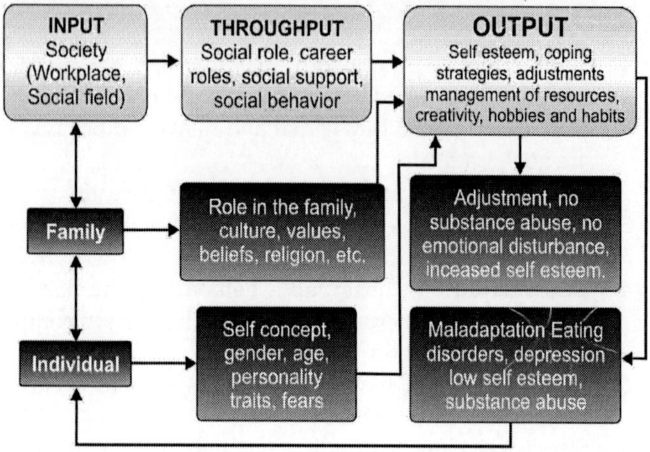

Fig. 3.3: Imogene King's theory of goal attainment for eating disorders

- The person is having a core that is protected by buffering systems.

Key Concepts

- **Central core:** The basic structure and energy reserves of the human that make life possible.
- **Flexible lines of defense:** Adaptive responses that fluctuate and protect the core from stressor penetration. Outermost line of defense.
- **Normal line of defense:** A conscious adaptation response usually used by an individual to protect the core from stressor penetration.
- **Lines of resistance:** Protection factors activated when stressors have penetrated the normal line of defence that are usually unconscious in nature.

Neuman's model focuses on stress reduction. It addresses how stress and individual response affects the development, maintenance and restoration of health.

- A person is a composite of psychologic, physiologic, sociocultural, developmental and spiritual variables that act harmoniously and simultaneously when encountered with stress from either the internal or external environments.
- Clients are persons, families, groups or communities who constantly interact with environment.

- Environment includes all internal and external factors or influences surrounding the client.
- **Internal environment:** Within the body.
- **The external environment:** Anything outside of the human body.
- **The created environment:** Individual perceptions of the internal and external environments.
- Stressors are tension-producing stimuli that have the potential to disturb a person's equilibrium.
- Stressors can be-intrapersonal, interpersonal or extra-personal.
- Stressors may by positive or negative.
- The basic structure and energy resources of humans need protection from encountered stressors.
- Reactions and resistance to stressors are provided by lines of defenses.
- Obvious reaction to stressor when lines of resistance are penetrated.
- The reaction may lead to restoration of balance or death.
- Three factors responsible for the person's reaction and recovery to encountered stressor are
  - The number and strength of the stressor.
  - The length of exposure to the stressor.
  - The meaningfulness of the stressor to the person.
- Newman defines illness as a state of insufficiency with disrupting needs unsatisfied.
- Nurses use primary, secondary or tertiary prevention to help clients attain optimal wellness.
- Model has wide application in nursing research (Fig. 3.4).
- Serves as a frame work for the WHO project "Nest of love" and for delivery of mental health services in Holland.

Person (A system): A composite of physiological, psychological, sociocultural, developmental and spiritual variables in interaction with the internal and external environment.

Environment: All internal and external factors of influences surrounding the client system.

Health: A continuum of wellness to illness

Nursing: Prevention as intervention.

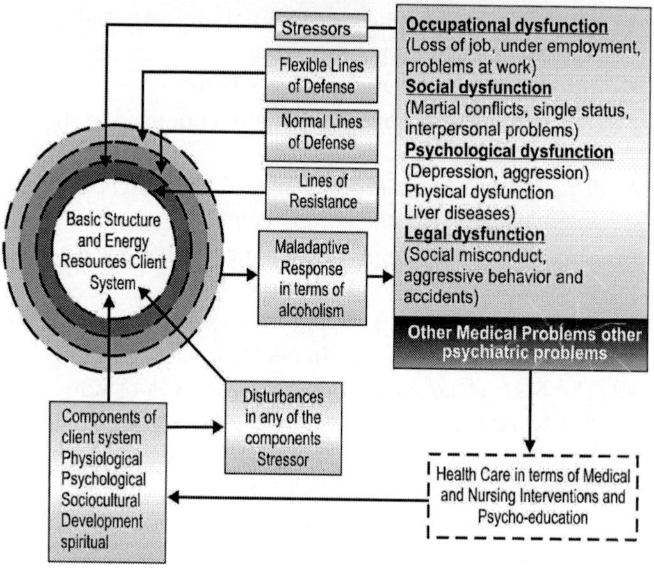

Fig. 3.4: Betty Neuman's theory application to alcoholism

CALISTA ROY'S ADAPTATION MODEL

- The stress/adaptation theory is the framework.
- The theory views change in terms of accommodation.
- People adjust to environmental changes to avoid disturbing a balanced existence.
- Provides a way to understand both how the balance is maintained and the possible effects of disturbed equilibrium.
- The theory is widely applied to explain, predict and control biologic responses of persons.
- It serves as traditional medical therapy.
- Compensation occurs constantly as the body adjusts to stimuli that tend to disturb equilibrium.
- A person's ability to adapt to changes in life events may determine the potential for health or disease.
- A person's reaction to stimuli involves cognitive appraisal and psychological coping methods in addition to physiologic reactions.

Sister Callista Roy's Adaptation Model

Person (human system): A whole with parts that function as a unity.

Environment: The world within and around humans as adaptive systems.

Health: A state and process of being and becoming an integrated and whole human being.

Nursing: Manipulation of stimuli to foster successful adaptation.

Calista Roy developed this model when she was confronted with the challenge of defining nursing as a PG nursing student.

The purpose of nursing is to promote a person's adaptation.

Adaptation is the process and outcome by which thinking and feeling persons use conscious awareness and choice to create human and environmental integration.

Key Concepts in Roy's Model

Stimulus: Point of interaction of the human system and environment. Stimulus produces a response.

Adaptive modes: Ways that a person adapts (through physiologic needs, self – concept, role function, interdependent relations)

Classes of stimuli: Focal, contextual and residual (non–specific stimuli, such as beliefs or attitudes). They may be equated with predisposing, precipitating and perpetuating factors responsible for the stressor to cause response in an individual.

Adaptation level: Range of a person's ability to adapt and create changes in the integrated, compensatory and compromised environments.

Coping: Ways of responding to the changing environment.

- The person as a unified system is a set of parts connected to function as a whole.
- The person constantly interacts with an ever-changing environment.
- The person's ability to respond positively reflects the level of adaptation.
- A focal stimuli is an environment change that requires an immediate adaptive response from the person.

- Contextual stimuli are all other stimuli present and accompany the focal stimuli.
- Residual stimuli mediate and contribute to the effect of focal stimulus.
- The combined effect of the three types of stimuli establishes the person's adaptation level.
- The person's adaptation level determines a zone that indicates the range of additional stimulation that will have a positive or adaptive response.
- If the stimulus crosses this adaptive zone then compromised adaptation ensues.
- Effective adaptation results in free energy available for use in subsequent adaptation to stimuli.
- Coping refers to routine, accustomed patterns of behaviors to deal with daily situations as well as to the production of new ways of behaving when drastic changes defeat the familiar responses.
- Two major coping mechanisms are regulator subsystem (biochemical responses) and the cognator subsystem (cognitive emotive channels)
- Four adaptive modes are physiologic—physical, self-concept-group identify, role function and interdependence.
- Desired result is a state in which conditions promote the person's goals, including survival, growth, reproduction, mastery and person and environment transformations.
- Health is viewed in light of human goals and the purposefulness of human existence.
- The goal of nursing is to promote adaptation by the use of nursing process, in each of the adaptive modes, thus contributing to health, quality of life and dying with dignity (Fig. 3.5).
- Any positive response by the person that creates free energy is considered as goal attainment.
- This free energy is used for responding to other stimuli.
- The goal of adaptation is fostered through nursing assessment and intervention, with the client as an active participant.
- Widely used for research.
- Provides a classification system for stimuli.

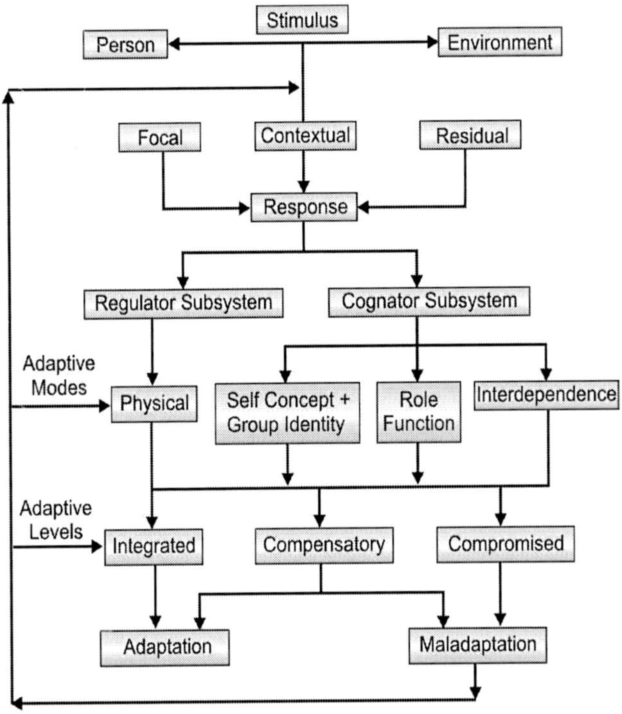

Fig. 3.5: Roy's stress/adaptation model

- Provides a system for classifying nursing assessment.
- Supports traditional practice of nursing.
- Used as a framework for nursing education for UG and PG nursing programs.
- Used as a foundation for health assessment in clinical practice.
- Provides guidance for nursing service.
- May be used by other health care professionals.

THE GROWTH MODEL OF CHANGE

It tends to focus on helping persons grow to realize and attain their full human potential. The caring theory or complexity theory is the basis for this model.

Caring Theory as A Framework

- Nursing practice focuses on caring for and about others.
- Caring are actions performed as well as concern demonstrated.
- Five categories of caring:
  - As a human trait
  - Moral imperative
  - Interpersonal relationship
  - Therapeutic intervention
  - As an affect.
- Client perceived caring as nursing ministrations that are person-centered, protective, anticipatory, physically comforting and that go beyond routine care.
- Nurses use psychosocial skills in caring along with professional competency.
- Caring outcomes are subjective experiences and objective client outcomes.
- Five caring processes:
  - Knowing
  - Being with
  - Doing for
  - Enabling
  - Maintaining belief.
- Five essences of caring with the other :
  - Interpersonal valuing and involvement.
  - Being there for and experiencing.
  - Instilling faith.
  - Concern and love for the other.
  - Actualization.

OREM'S SELF-CARE DEFICIT THEORY

- The purpose of nursing is to help people meet their self care needs.
- Nurses do for others what they cannot do for themselves.

Key Concepts

- **Self-care:** Learned behaviors that a person performs for self that contribute to health.

- **Self-care deficit:** A relationship between actions a person should take for healthy functioning and the capability for action.
- **Self-care requisites:** Needs that are universal or associated with development or deviation from health.
- **Self-care demand:** Therapeutic actions to meet needs.
- **Agency:** Capability to engage in self-care.
- **Person (Patient):** A person under care of a nurse.
- **Environment:** Physical, chemical, biologic and social contexts within which human beings exist.
- **Health:** A state characterized by soundness or wholeness of developed human structures and of bodily and mental functioning.
- **Nursing:** Actions to overcome or prevent the development of a self–care deficit or provides therapeutic self-care for a patient who is unable to do so.

Orem's Three-part Nursing Theory

- The theory focuses on persons in relations.
- The theory of self-care focuses on the self, the I.
- The theory of self care deficit focuses on you and me.
- The theory of nursing systems focuses on we, the persons in community.
- Self-care is defined as the voluntary regulation of one's own human functioning and development that is necessary for individuals to maintain life, health, wellbeing.
- People learn self-care activities as they mature.
- Self-care activities are influenced by culture, society, family customs, age, developmental state and health status.
- Nursing care is concerned with the person's need for self-care to sustain life and health, recover from disease or injury and cope with their effects.
- Health is physical, physiological and mental functioning of developed human structures.
- Health is a state of wholeness or integrity of human beings.
- Individuals move toward maturation and achieve human potential.
- Self care requisites due to development or health deviations.

Universal self-care Requisites

- Maintenance of sufficient air, water and food intake.
- Provision of care associated with elimination processes and excrements.
- Maintenance of a balance between activity and rest and between solitude and special interaction.
- Prevention of hazards to life, functioning and wellbeing.
- Promotion of human functioning and development within social groups in accord with potential, known limitations and the desire to be normal.

Therapeutic Self-care Demands are Determined by—

- Identifying existing or potential self-care requisites.
- Developing methods for meeting self-care requisites.
- Designing, implementing and evaluating a plan of action.

Nursing process is used as a way to develop a system of nursing.

Self-care Deficit Theory Promotes Care at Following Levels—

- Fully compensatory care.
- Partially compensatory care.
- Supportive educative care.

Nursing interventions are aimed at maintaining health, preventing illness and restoring health.

Uses

- Nurses use nursing process and specifically focus on interventions and implementation of nursing interventions.
- Widely used in practice and education.
- Widely used in nursing research of descriptive nature.
- Categorizes clients and health agency as self care agency, dependent care and dependent care agency.
- Promotes progressive patient care concept and quality assured care.

Complexity Theory as a Framework

- Assumes that the reality continuously changes.
- Change is irregular and cannot be predicted.

- Emphasizes change over time, long-term unpredictability and openness to the environment with mutual simultaneous interactions.
- Other assumptions include patterns mutual, simultaneous interactions continual fluctuations that reveal variable patterns.

Critical Points

- The whole cannot be known from the sum of the parts nor can the sum of parts be more than the whole because everything is unitary.
- Emphasizes becoming of the human being in terms of potential for change.
- Found difficult to understand as it challenges to think in multiple dimensions.

MARTHA ROGER'S SCIENCE OF UNITARY BEINGS

- Developed while searching for a specific and unique body of knowledge for nursing.
- The purpose of nursing is to foster health potential.

Key Concepts

- **Unitary human being:** An irreducible, indivisible, pandimensional energy field identified by pattern.
- **Unified energy field:** A pandimensional nonlinear domain without special or temporal attributes.
- **Mutual process:** Changes within the human and environmental fields that occur simultaneously.
- **Person (human being):** A unitary energy field with a unique pattern.
- **Environment:** An energy field in mutual process with the human being.
- **Health:** An indication of the complexity and innovative patterning of the energy field that is the person.
- **Nursing:** Intervening to improve pattern manifestations and the environment to achieve maximum health potentials.

The person as a unified energy field continuously exchanges energy with an environmental energy field. Man is unified, possesses his own integrity and manifests characteristics that are more than and different from the sum of his parts.

- It is impossible to describe human by combining attributes of each of the parts. Only when any of the part lose its identity, it is possible to describe the person.
- Parts of human whole include, physical, biological, psychological, social, cultural, spiritual attributes that are merged together in an invisible whole.
- Changes are due to interactions of energy fields of human and environment.
- These changes bring about complexity and innovativeness of the person.
- Each person is unique.
- Changes are irreversible and unidirectional spiral with self regulation and directed toward achieving increasing complexity of organization.
- The person is characterized by the capacity for abstraction, imagery, language and thought, sensation and emotion.
- Nursing intervention is aimed toward promoting the betterment of humans.
- Caring in nursing is a way of using knowledge.

Three Principles of Change

- **Integrality:** Human and environment must be perceived simultaneously.
- **Helicy:** Continuous, innovative, unpredictable, diverse change.
- **Resonancy:** Change occurs from lower frequency longer waver patterns to higher frequency, shorter wave patterns.

Understanding of the mechanisms that affect the life process in human is vital. This knowledge aids nurses to purposefully intervene. The change is in the health status for the client and in the nurse too.

Uses

- For future theory development that to be used in practice.
- Science of unitary human beings as a foundation for practice.
- Theory of power based on this unitary science is used in nursing service administration.

- Widely used in research.
- Used as a foundation in validating effectiveness of complementary and alternative health practices.

ROSEMARIE PARSE'S HUMAN BECOMING THEORY

- Purpose of nursing is to improve the quality of life for both the client and nurse.

Key Concepts

- **Constitution:** Development of patterning through person-environment interaction.
- **Coexistence:** Dynamic mutual processes between the person and the environment.
- **Situated freedom:** Freedom of choice in a situation.
- **Person:** An open being, more than and different from the sum of parts.
- **Environment:** In mutual process with the person.
- **Health:** Continuously changing process of becoming.
- **Nursing:** Use of true presence to facilitate the becoming of the participant.
- The emphasis is on the meaning and values that influence a person's active choices of behavior.
- The person constructs his or her own meaning.
- Health is a nonlinear entity and incorporates values.
- As a person interacts with the environment, patterns of relating are established.
- These provide insight into person's patterning and values at that moment.
- The nurse's goal is to be truly present with the people as they enhance their quality of life.
- **Key processes in the model are—**

– Imaging	– Transforming
– Valuing	– Originating
– Languaging	– Revealing
– Connecting	– Enabling
– Powering	– limiting

- The meaning of human beliefs and values is developed and demonstrated through words and movement.
- Human patterns in relating to others are derived from multiple choices and involve rhythmical processes of moving closer to and away from others.
- It involves the processes of distancing and moving closer in interrelationships that provide the force for change and creativity.
- The unitary human freely chooses meaning in situation, bears responsibility for the choices and transcends with possible.

Three Implications for Practice

- Illuminating meaning by explicating what is appearing through language.
- Synchronizing rhythms by dwelling with the flow of connecting separating.
- Mobilizing transcendence by moving towards possible in transforming.

Living the belief system is through true presence which is a non-routinized, unconditional loving way. The nurse witnesses the blossoming of others. The nurse is an empathetic sounding board for client and families to express their feelings and concerns. The process of expression is through language and movement.

The nurse connects with clients through focused interactions rather than doing things for them. A phenomenological – hermeneutic methodology to test relationships depicted in the model is suggested by Parse.

Uses

- Conceptual frame work for research.
- Emphasizes the importance of meaning that underlies behavior.
- Provides a structure for the identification and clarification of manifestations.
- Useful for practice that includes multidimensional client healing, enhanced personal growth and continued professional growth.

MARGARET NEWMAN'S THEORY OF HEALTH AS EXPANDING CONSCIOUSNESS

According to Margaret Newman:

- The purpose of nursing is to promote a higher level of consciousness in both client and nurse (Fig. 3.6).
- Consciousness is the capacity of the system to interact with its environment, the informational capacity of the system.
- The focus of nursing is the pattern of the whole, health as pattern of the evolving whole, with caring as a moral imperative.
- Health is viewed as a process that encompasses both disease and non disease.
- Disease is a meaningful component of the whole and a possible facilitator of health.
- The task for nursing intervention is to recognize patterning and relate to it in an authentic way.

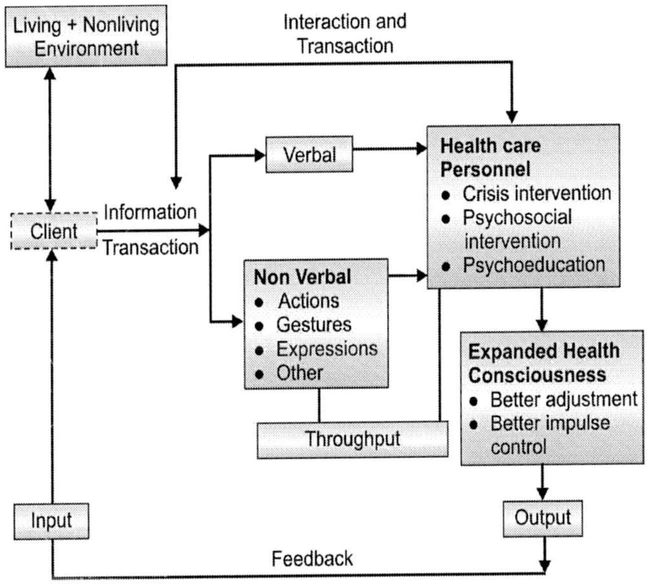

Fig. 3.6: Margaret Newman's theory of health as expanding consciousness

Major Concepts

- **Person (human being):** Unitary and continuous with the undivided wholeness of the universe.
- **Environment:** Undivided wholeness of the universe.
- **Health:** Expansion of consciousness.
- **Nursing:** Facilitating representating of the client to higher levels of consciousness.

Uses

- Contributes to the body of knowledge about healthy patterning of unitary human beings.
- Describes a methodology for research.
- Widely used by researches.

Nursing theories are the evolving concept in nursing. They are applied to nursing practice and problems of nurse clinicians. They have implications in nursing education, nursing administration and nursing service-practice. More and more nurse researchers need to use them and emerge with new ones that would improve nursing knowledge and practice.

CHAPTER

4

Ethical Issues in Research

Although guidelines that govern human behavior have always been a part of recorded history, the need for ethical standards in research came to the public's attention in a dramatic way following World War II when evidence of the Nazi's experimentation and torture of selected groups of victims was revealed.

- Ethical issues are prominent in nursing research because of blurring of the line of demarcation between the collection of research information and the expected practice of nursing.
- Ethical challenges increase with the need to produce evidence of the highest possible quality for practice.
- Ethical issues are not given adequate attention all the times.

MAIN ISSUES OF CONCERN

- No intervention to some of the participants.
- Research intervention administered without consent of the participants.
- Deliberate harm or discomfort.
- Inadequate confidentiality.
- Misuse of research information.

CODE OF ETHICS

Code of ethics is developed to protect human rights.

- Nuremberg code developed after Nazi atrocities.
- Declaration of Helsinki adopted in 1964 by World Medical Association and revised in 2000.
- Indian Council for Medical Research (ICMR) Guidelines to be followed in India.
- Belmont report 1978 serves as the basis for regulations affecting research.

ARTICLES ADAPTED FROM THE NUREMBERG CODE

- The voluntary consent of human subjects is absolutely necessary.
- The experiment should yield fruitful results for the good of society.
- The experiment should be so designed and based on results of animal experimentation and knowledge of the disease or problem under study that the anticipated results will justify performance of the experiment.
- The experiment should be conducted so as to avoid all unnecessary physical and mental suffering and harm.
- No experiment should be conducted where there is a prior reason to believe that death or injury will occur.
- The degree of risk should never exceed than determined benefit of the importance of the problem to be solved by the experiment.
- Proper preparations should be made to protect the experimental subject against even remote possibilities of injury, disability, or death.
- Scientifically qualified people must only conduct the experiment. The highest degree of skill and care should be required through all stages of the experiment.
- During the course of the experiment, the subject should be at liberty to bring the experiment to an end.
- During the course of the experiment, the scientist must be prepared to terminate the experiment at any stage.

ETHICAL DILEMMAS

Some dilemmas occur out of a conviction that knowledge is important and potentially life saving or beneficial to others in the long run.

Participants' rights and study demands are put in direct conflict.

- The participants' usual behavior is altered because of the known presence of research observers thus questioning the validity of the findings.
- Probing for information could be painful and even traumatic for the participants.

- Potential hazards of the untested intervention in terms of side effects.
- Some participant's denied of benefits of intervention (control group).
- Close involvement of researcher with the participants may reveal illegal or immoral behavior of the participant posing questions to confidentiality.

ETHICAL PRINCIPLES

Beneficence

Most fundamental ethical principles in research is that of beneficence, which imposes a duty on research to minimize harm and to maximize benefits.

The Right to Freedom from Harm and Discomfort

- Researchers have an obligation to avoid, prevent or minimize harm in studies with humans.
- Participants are not to be subjected to unnecessary risk for harm or discomfort.
- Participation must be essential to achieve scientifically and socially important aims that could not otherwise be realized.
- Harm and discomfort can be physical, emotional, social, or financial.
- Strategies to minimize all types of harms and discomfort, even temporary ones.
- Research to be done by qualified people.
- Researcher to be prepared to discontinue study in case of suspect of injury, death, disability or undue distress to study participants.
- Prior studies with tissue cultures and animals before proceeding with human subjects.
- Close attention to the psychological consequences of intervention to participants.

The Right to Protection from Exploitation

- The study participants should not be at a disadvantage or exposed to the situations for which they are not prepared.

- Assurance that information from them will never be used against them in any way.
- The special relationship between the researcher and participants is crucial and not to be exploited.

Respect for Human Dignity

Respect for human dignity is the second ethical principle in the Belmont report. It includes the right to self-determination and the right to full disclosure.

The Right to Self-determination

- Humans are autonomous agents capable of controlling their own activities.
- Self-determination means participants right to decide voluntarily whether to participate in a study, without risking any penalty or prejudicial treatment.
- The right to ask questions
- To refuse to give information.
- To withdraw from the study.

  Coercion: Explicit and Implicit threats of penalty for failing to participate in a study or excessive rewards from agreeing to participate.
- Researcher is in a position of authority, control or influence over potential participants.

The Right to Full Disclosure

- People's right to make informed, voluntary decisions about study participation, which require full disclosure.
- Full disclosure means the researcher has to fully describe the nature of the study, the person's right to refuse participation, the researcher's responsibilities, likely risks and benefits.
- The right is a major element of informed consent.
- Full disclosure creates two types of biases: (i) Biases from inaccurate data. (ii) Bias from sampling recruitment problems. This undermines the study.
- Hence covert data collection, deception techniques are used.

Justice

It includes participants' right to fair treatment and right to privacy.

The Right to Fair Treatment

Justice connotes fairness and equity.

- There should be equitable distribution of benefits and burdens of research.
- No vulnerable or compromised candidates to be study participants.
- Obligations towards individuals who are unable to protect their own interests.
- Nobody to be exploited for the advancement of knowledge.
- Duty to neither neglect nor discriminate against the beneficiaries of research.
- Selection of study participants based on research requirements.
- Non prejudicial treatment to non-participants.
- Sensitivity to and respect for the beliefs, habits, lifestyles of people from different backgrounds or cultures.
- Provide required clarifications.
- Courteous and factual treatment to the participants.

Right to Privacy

- All research involves intruding into personal lives.
- Participant's privacy is maintained throughout the study.
- Data provided by participants to be kept in strictest confidence.
- Standards to protect patient's medical records and other health information to be followed.

The ethical issues for the novice researchers may be challenging and demotivating at times. To overcome such distressing feelings and prevent resulting dislike for the research; always do the following:

- Have the research proposal approved by the Institutional Review Board.
- Take informed consent from every subject.
- Maintain information regarding confidentiality and anonymity.
- Be extracareful when using vulnerable subjects.

- Evaluate whether the potential benefits of participation outweigh the possible risks.
- Clarify all the doubts of the participants before recruiting them for the study.
- Inform the participants how they can access the results of the study.

Thus ethical issues are the guards against the misuse of subjects, information by the researcher(s). Nurses very often conduct research on vulnerable population like pregnant women, children of school age, adolescents and mentally ill clients. Extra precautions are required to be taken to maintain their confidentiality to prevent defamation and misuse of their information by third party payers, family members, relatives and employers of the subjects.

CHAPTER 5

Research Designs

The word design implies both creativity and structure. The design for a research study can be seen as a road map or a recipe. It serves as a fairly flexible set of guidelines that will provide the searcher with answers to the questions of inquiry.

To choose a research design, the nurse must first develop a vision of the overall plan for a study, including a general idea of the type of data needed to answer the research question. The design is a critical link that connects the researcher's framework with appropriate types of data. The level of pre-existing knowledge in the area of inquiry also helps determine the research design.

TYPES OF RESEARCH

See Figures 5.1 and 5.2.

CHARACTERISTICS OF QUANTITATIVE STUDIES

Quantitative studies are undertaken to establish causality among the variables.

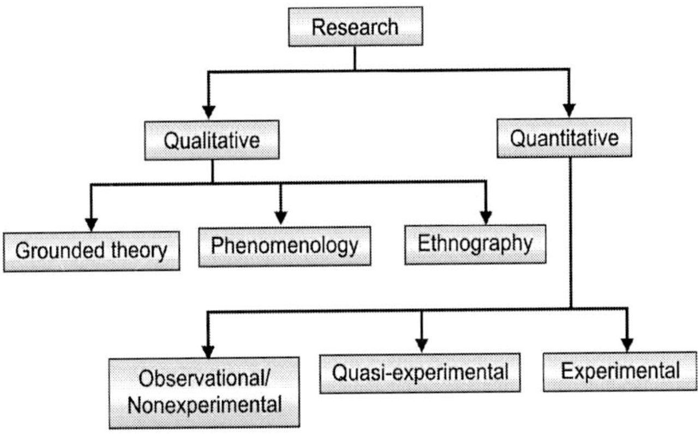

Fig. 5.1: Research designs

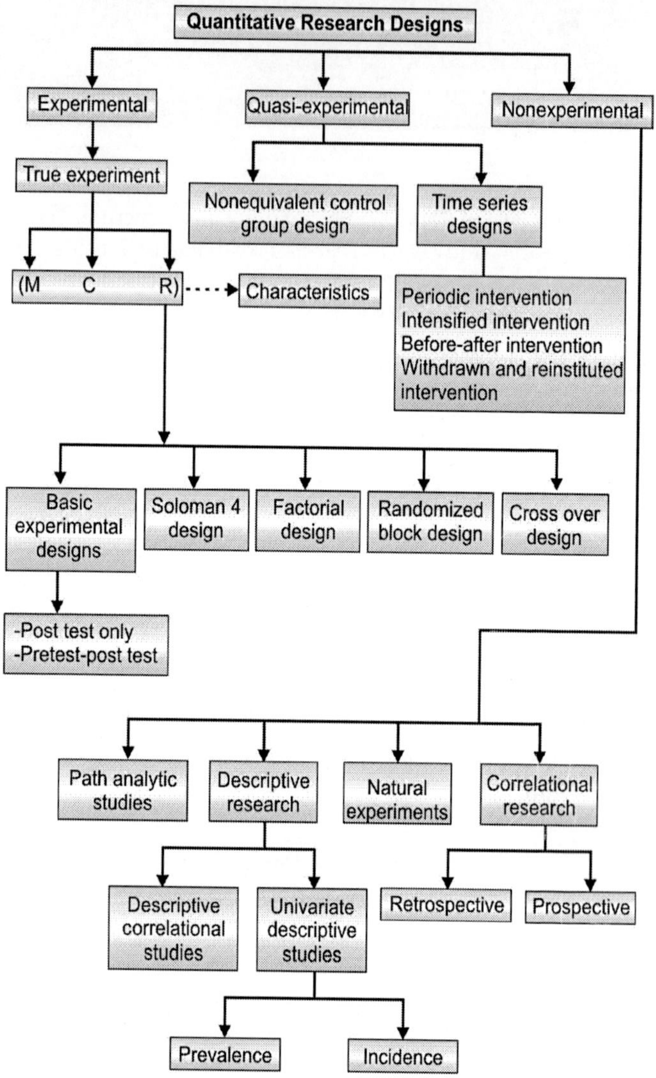

Fig. 5.2: Quantitative research designs

Causality: A study of quantitative nature that yields the strongest possible evidence to answer the research question. Many research questions are causes and effects, e.g. high caloric intake causes weight gain

- Most causes in which health researchers are interested are not deterministic. They only increase the chance that an effect will occur, e.g. smoking is a cause of lung cancer but not everyone who smokes develops lung cancer and not everyone with lung cancer is a smoker.

THE COUNTER FACTUAL MODEL

In a research context, a counterfactual is what would have happened to the same people exposed to a causal factor if they simultaneously were not exposed to the causal factor.

- An effect represents the difference between what actually did happen with the exposure and what would have happened without it.
- It is a good model, an ideal one to provide evidence about causes and effects.

Criteria for Causality

- **Temporal relationship:** A cause must precede an effect in time.
- **Empirical relationship:** There has to be logical relationship between the presumed cause and the presumed effect.
- The relationship between the cause and effect cannot be explained as being caused by a third variable. (The relationship is absolutely between the cause and effect and no third party interferes in the relationship).
- **Coherence:** Similar evidence is obtained from multiple sources.
- **Consistency:** Similar levels of statistical relationship in several studies.
- **Biologic plausibility:** Evidence from laboratory or basic physiologic studies showing that a causal pathway is credible.

Experimental Design

- The experimental design is also called randomized controlled trial – RCT.

  The researchers are active agents and not passive observers in this.
- Mere observation is valuable but the complexities occurring in nature often make it difficult to understand important relationships.

- This problem is handled by isolating the phenomena in a laboratory and controlling the conditions under which they occurred.
- The controlled experiment is considered as the gold standard for yielding reliable evidence about causes and effects.
- The strength of true experiment lies in the fact that experimenter achieves greater confidence in the genuineness of causal relationships as they are observed under controlled conditions.
- True experiments offer the most convincing evidence about the effect one variable has on another.

PROPERTIES OF RCT

Manipulation: Also called intervention or treatment that the experimenter introduces to at least some subjects.

Control: The experimenter exerts control over the experimental situation called a control group/arm that does not receive the intervention. In some studies, alternative or some standard treatment may be given to one group.

Randomization: The experimenter assigns subjects to a control or experimental condition on a random basis.

MANIPULATION

Manipulation involves doing something to study participants. The experimenter manipulates the independent variable by administering a treatment (intervention) to some subjects. The intervention is not administered to the other remaining subjects. The remaining subjects may be given some other treatment. Thus the independent variable is varied deliberately and the effect on the dependent variable is observed.

Manipulation can be done in two ways as under -

1. Manipulation of the experimental intervention.
2. Manipulation of the control condition.

Manipulation of the Experimental Intervention

In this, the manipulation is done with the experimental intervention. This means an identical treatment/intervention for all subjects in the treatment group or group under study; or

- The intervention is tailored to fit the individual subjects need.
- Tailored interventions are more effective than standardized interventions.
- 'What' works is equally important 'what works for whom.' Thus the researchers must delineate the full nature of intervention clearly. This should answer following questions–
  - What is the intervention?
  - What are the alternative interventions?
  - How do the alternative interventions differ from one, selected for study?
  - What are specific procedures to be used for the intervention?
  - What is the dosage/intensity of the intervention?
  - How long the intervention to be administered?
  - Who will administer the intervention?
  - What type of training to be given to the implementers?
  - Under what conditions the interventions to be withdrawn or altered?

Manipulation of the Control Condition

- Obtaining evidence about relationships requires making at least one comparison.
- The term control group refers to a group of subjects whose performance on a dependent variable is used to evaluate the performance of treatment group on the same dependent variable.
- In medical research, the control group or condition is denoted by the term control arm.
- The control group condition represents a proxy for the ideal counterfactual.
- The manipulation of the control arm can be as follows :
  - Control group subjects receive no intervention.
  - Control group subjects receive alternative intervention.
  - Control group subjects receive placebo-pseudo intervention which is presumed to have no therapeutic value.
  - Control group subjects receive different doses of the treatment as compared to experimental group subjects who receive richer or more intense and longer intervention.
  - Control group is a wait list control group with delayed treatment which is eventually full treatment.

- Methodologically, the best possible test is between two conditions that are extremes like experimental group received the intervention and control group get no treatment/ intervention.
- Ethically, the most appealing counterfactual is the wait list/ delay of intervention approach.

RANDOMIZATION

- Also called as random assignment or random allocation.
- It involves placing subjects into treatment conditions at random.
- Random means every subject has an equal chance of being assigned to any group.

Principles of Randomization

- The overall purpose of randomization is to approximate the ideal but impossible counterfactual of having the same people in multiple treatment groups simultaneously.
- Although randomization is for equalizing groups there is no guarantee that the groups will, in fact, be equal.
- The likelihood of obtaining markedly unequal groups is reduced as the number of subjects increase.
- With randomization, all possible distinctive characteristics are likely to be equally distributed in all groups.
- Randomization is the most trustworthy and acceptable method of equalizing groups, as it provides statistical reliability to the study.

Randomization Procedures

- Randomization depends on the allocation process which should be random and unbiased, and there must be strict adherence to the resulting randomization schedule.
- Random assignment should involve allocation concealment that prevents the enrolled subjects from knowing the upcoming assignments.
- Allocation information by telephone or e-mail can be employed. The employing person is unconnected with recruitment, enrollment or treatment.

- Eligibility for the study should be ascertained before randomization.
- Randomization should occur as closely as possible to the start of the intervention.
- Procedures of randomization include
  - Head or tails coin tossing.
  - Telephone or e-mail by unconnected person.
  - Using table of random numbers.
- Baseline data of subjects must be collected before enrollment of subject for the experiment.

Randomization Variants

Randomization involves the random assignment of individual subjects to different conditions.

1. **Cluster Randomization:** Involves randomly assigning clusters of individuals to different treatment groups.

   This enhances the feasibility of conducting a true experiment.

   This approach also reduces the possibility of contamination of treatments. (Mingling of subjects in the groups which could cloud the results due to exchange of information).

   The main disadvantage is that the data obtained are more complex, and sample size requirements are usually greater for a given level of accuracy.

   The complexity of data makes the research synthesis complicated.
2. **Stratification:** Involves subgrouping of study participants in equal sizes to allocate the treatment conditions.
3. **Permuted block randomization:** Involves random allocation for block of subjects of even size instead of randomization for the entire sample.
   - Random assignment with the small block would guarantee an appropriate distribution across conditions.
   - This is useful when enrollment occurs over a long period of time and when there are chances that enrolling technique or the intervention itself may change due to improved proficiency in the implementation.
4. **Randomized consent:** It is the full information being given to the subjects about the intervention and the study purpose.

- Randomization may be done after obtaining the fully informed consent from the subjects.
  The subjects may opt out of study due to this. Hence subjects may be randomized before obtaining the informed consent from them.
- Partially randomized patient preference approach includes asking preferences of the study participants about treatment conditions. Here only those without a strong preference are randomized but all the subjects are followed up.

Masking or Blinding

- This is allocation concealment.
- It is intended to prevent biases that could result from foreknowledge of allocations.
- It can be implemented in all conditions irrespective of the intervention.
- Biases could be —
  - Researcher's awareness of who is in which treatment condition.
  - Participant's awareness of intervention that may bring about certain behavioral changes irrespective of the treatment.
- Masking of the treatment status of subjects from the people collecting outcome data is always desirable and possible.

TYPES OF EXPERIMENTAL RESEARCH DESIGNS

Basic experimental designs: There are two types of basic research designs. They are:

a. **After only design or a posttest design:** In this, the data on dependent variable is collected only once after random assignment is completed and the experimental treatment is introduced.

   — X O

   X is intervention and O is observation or data collected after the intervention.

b. **Before-after design or pretest–posttest design:** In this, the dependent variable is measured twice, before and after the intervention. It is the most commonly used design. Researchers can examine change due to intervention.

O_1	X	O_2
Pretest	Intervention	Posttest

Solomon four group design: In this, the pretest and posttest data are collected for both, the experimental group as well as control group. There are four groups; namely, two experimental groups and two control groups. Pretest data are collected for each of control and experimental group. Control group is not administered the intervention.

Experimental group with pretest	O_1	X	O_2
Experimental group without pretest	—	X	O_2
Control group with pretest	O_1	—	O_2
Control group without pretest	—	—	O_2

Factorial design: Factorial design takes into consideration two or more variables simultaneously. It addresses three or more research questions. The strength of factorial design is that it permits us to evaluate not only main effects but also interaction effects. In this, the studies are assigned at random to a specific combination of conditions. It can be performed with three or more independent variables.

The independent variables are called factors. Two therapeutic strategies can be studied. It helps to test multiple hypotheses in a single experiment. It compares between the hypotheses having effect on dependent variable. One of the factors can be considered as independent variable.

Time	*Treatment – I* A_1	*Treatment – II* A_2	*Treatment I + II* $A_1 + A_2 = A_3$
30 minutes –B_1	$A_1 B_1$	$A_2 B_1$	$A_3 B_1$
60 minutes – B_2	$A_1 B_2$	$A_2 B_2$	$A_3 B_2$

Randomized block design: In this design, there are two factors (independent variables), but one factor is not experimentally manipulated and the other factor is a stratifying variable. The variable gender cannot be manipulated and hence blocked or is a stratifying variable. Similarly, age can be a stratifying variable.

The design is similar to factorial design. It permits examination of interaction effects. It can be extended to include more than one blocking variable. More than one manipulating variable can be included. It enhances the researchers control over the composition of samples. Here one group acts as a control for the other.

Treatment/Intervention	*Treatment 1A_1*	*Treatment 2A_2*
Male – B_1	$A_1 B_1$	$A_2 B_1$
Female – B_2	$A_1 B_2$	$A_2 B_2$

Cross-over design: A cross-over design involves the exposure of the same subjects to more than one experimental treatment. Advantage of ensuring the highest possible equivalence among subjects exposed to different conditions. The groups are equal with respect to age, weight, health and so on. That means the groups are homogenous groups. When there are three or more conditions to which each subject will be exposed, the procedure of counterbalancing can be used to rule out ordering effects.

It is an extremely powerful design at times. There may be problem of carry over effects which may interfere with inferences.

MCR is present and the subjects serve as their own controls.

A	B	C	A	C	B
B	C	A	B	A	C
C	A	B	C	B	A

Strengths of Experiments

- Controlled experiments are often the ideal of science.
- Most powerful method to test hypothesis of cause and effect relationships between variables.
- Considered as gold standard for intervention studies as it yields the highest quality evidence regarding intervention's effect.
- Randomization and use of comparison conditions makes it attain ideal counterfactual status.
- Causal relationship can be inferred with confidence.
- Alternative explanations to a causal interpretation, is ruled out due to use of manipulation, comparison and randomization.
- Meta-analysis of RCTs provides rich evidence for questions related to causes.

- Double blind RCTs are very powerful where the participants and implementers are unaware of their roles the studies.

Limitations of Experiments

- Sometimes they are criticized for artificiality.
- Difficulty in randomization may be present because in ordinary life, people's interactions are not random.
- Focus is on only a handful of variables while holding all else constant.
- Treatment or intervention is by the people not in the research team. Hence, the implementation may not be adequate, satisfactory or as it should have been.
- It is difficult to maintain the integrity of intervention and control conditions if the study period extends over time.
- Study may be conducted in clinical settings over which researchers have little or no control.
- The intervention may be diluted through non-participation making the interpretation difficult.
- The Hawthorn effect or placebo effect due to people's expectations may be present.
- Subjects might be aware of their participation and might alter their actions accordingly.

QUASI-EXPERIMENTS

Quasi-experiments involve an intervention but lack randomization. Some quasi-experiments even lack a control group. The signature of a quasi-experimental design is an intervention in the absence of randomization. Quasi-experiments are not powerful in establishing causal relationship between interventions and outcomes.

Types of Quasi-experimental Designs

Nonequivalent Control Group designs

This is the most frequently used quasi-experimental design. It involves an experimental treatment and two groups of subjects observed before and after its implementation.

Symbolically it is represented as:

E – O_1 X O_2

C – O_1 X O_2

The subjects are not randomly assigned to treatment groups. The design is weaker because it can no longer be assumed that the experimental and comparison groups are equivalent at the outset. The design is strong because the baseline data allow us to determine whether the subjects in two groups had similar satisfaction initially. If the comparison and experimental groups are similar at baseline, the posttest results could be confidently inferring causal relationship.

The term comparison group is synonym of control group against which outcomes in the experimental group are evaluated. The non-equivalent control group after only design is pre-experimental and is denoted as:

E -	X	O
C -	—	O

The use of matching ensures that the groups are equivalent on at least some key variables related to the outcomes. This can be an improvement in the standard before-after nonequivalent control group design. Two or more samples from different locations may be included in the study.

Time Series Designs

In this design, there is no randomization and no control. The only kind of comparison that can be made is a before-after contrast.

The design has the weakness as it cannot control external factors that may influence the outcomes. The design gives significant relationship in certain cases where pre and posttest data are collected immediately before and after the intervention. In a time series design, information is collected over an extended period and an intervention is introduced during that period.

The extended time period strengthens the ability to attribute change to the intervention.

- One group before-after time series design
  Intervention
  O_1 X O_2
  One group single observation before-after
  O_1 O_2 O_3 O_4 X O_5 O_6 O_7 O_8
- One group multiple observations before-after time series

It permits to rule out the possibility that the data reflect unstable measurement at one point.

- A powerful quasi-experiment design is a combination of the time series and nonequivalent control group designs.

  Numerous variations on the simple time series are possible and are being used by nurse researchers.

  $O_1 \quad O_2 \quad O_3 \quad O_4 \quad X \quad O_5 \quad O_6 \quad O_7 \quad O_8 - E$

  $O_1 \quad O_2 \quad O_3 \quad O_4 \quad - \quad O_5 \quad O_6 \quad O_7 \quad O_8 - C$

  Two group multiple observations before-after time series

- Additional evidence regarding the effects of a treatment can be achieved by instituting the treatment at several points in time.

  $O_1 \quad O_2 \quad X \quad O_3 \quad O_4 \quad X \quad O_5 \quad O_6 \quad X \quad O_7 \quad O_8$

- Strengthening the treatment over time.

  $O_1 \quad O_2 \quad X \quad O_3 \quad O_4 \quad X+1 \quad O_5 \quad O_6 \quad X+2 \quad O_7 \quad O_8$

- Instituting the treatment at one point in time, then withdrawing the treatment at a later point, sometimes reinstituting the treatment again.

  $O_1 \quad O_2 \quad X \quad O_3 \quad O_4 \quad (-X) \quad O_5 \quad O_6 \quad X \quad O_7 \quad O_8$

These designs are typically longitudinal designs. Most often used for policy making. One of the shortcoming is non-adherence to the intervention by the subjects. Possible in real life settings and practical when true experiment is not possible. Outcomes are not very reliable. Cause and effect interferences are less convincing. Several rival hypotheses come up that compete with the experimental manipulation.

Single Subject Experiments

They use time series designs to gather information about an intervention based on the responses of a single subject under controlled conditions.

Regression Discontinuity Design

It involves systematic assignment of subjects to groups based on cut-off scores on a pre-intervention measure.

Those with preference are given the conditions they prefer and are followed up as part of the study.

They provide valuable information about the subjects' preference of one condition over other.

The weakness due to heterogeneous group conditions may interfere with influences. This design is rarely used by nurse researchers.

Dose Response Design

In this, the outcomes of those receiving different doses of a treatment are compared. Some subjects may attend more sessions or get more intensive treatment than others. The outcome is always not directly proportional to the interventions. Differences in motivation, physical function and other characteristics of subjects could interfere with the outcome.

It may establish a causal inference when comparison is within an experiment.

Strengths of Quasi-experiments

- They are practical.
- They introduce some research control when true experiment is not possible.
- People are unwilling for randomization and control hence quasi-experiments are better suited than true experiments. They have implications for the generalizability of results.

Limitations of Quasi-experiments

- Results are less conclusive.
- Researchers must be aware of the weakness of quasi-experiments in order to counteract at least those weaknesses that interfere with the results.
- Rival hypotheses compete with experimental manipulation as explanations for the results.
- Conclusions are dependent in part on human judgement and hence cause-effect inferences are less convincing.

NONEXPERIMENTAL RESEARCH DESIGNS

When researchers do not intervene by manipulating the independent variable, the study is nonexperimental or observational. Most of the nursing research is observational. Birth weight, body temperature, ethnicity, etc. are the characteristics that cannot be manipulated experimentally. Some variables may be technically manipulated but not ethically, e.g. prenatal care. Non-experimental research is usually needed before an experimental study.

Types of Nonexperimental Research Designs

Correlational Designs

In this design, the researchers study the effect of a potential cause that they cannot manipulate and examine the relationship between variables.

Correlation means association between two variables. Variation in one has a tendency of variation in another, e.g. taller people have more weight than shorter ones.

It is risky to infer causal relationship in correlational research because of lack of control over the independent variable and absence of an ideal counterfactual. The independent variable has usually already occurred in the past.

a. Retrospective Designs

It is also called as case control study design. In this design, a presently existing phenomena is linked to phenomena that occurred in the past, before the study was initiated. The researcher is interested in a present outcome and attempts to determine antecedent factors that caused it, e.g. smoking linked to lung cancer.

The case control studies begin with group of people who are cases and another group called control. It is going back in time. The research begins with dependent variable and then examines whether it is correlated with one or more antecedent independent variables.

Often cross-sectional design with data on both the dependent and independent variables are collected once.

It can demonstrate comparability between cases and controls.

Inferences regarding the presumed cause of the disease are enhanced. Difficulty is due to the groups which are almost never totally comparable with respect to all potential factors influencing the dependent variable. This approach is used to identify risk factors for different problems or conditions where the outcome is the degree/amount of some condition.

b. Prospective Nonexperimental Design

A nonexperimental prospective study starts with a presumed cause and then goes forward in time to the presumed effect. It is also called cohort study. Prospective studies are more costly. They are longitudinal in nature requiring a substantial follow-up period. Steps are to be taken to confirm that all subjects are free from the effect at the time the independent variable is measured. To rule out the existence of effect may be difficult and costly at times, e.g. lung cancer may be present but not yet diagnosed at the time of recruitment of the subject in the study.

Prospective studies are stronger that retrospective studies. Samples are more likely to be representative. Investigators may impose controls to rule out competing explanations for the results. Some prospective studies are exploratory. Sometimes, they are accused of as going on "fishing expeditions."

Natural Experiments

In this design, a group exposed to natural or other phenomena is compared with a non-exposed group. The researcher does not intervene here. The independent variable need not be a 'natural' phenomenon. It could be fire, lottery win, floods, terrorist attack etc. If pre-intervention measures are available, before-after comparisons are profitable in natural experiments.

Path Analytic Studies

Researchers interested in testing theories of causation based on nonexperimental data through causal chain among a set of independent variables, mediating variables and a dependent variable. This allows researcher to test whether non-experimental data conform sufficiently to the underlying model to justify causal inferences.

Descriptive Research Designs

The purpose of descriptive studies is to observe, describe and document aspects of a situation, as it naturally occurs and sometimes to serve as a starting point for hypothesis generation or theory development.

a. *Descriptive Correlational Research*

To describe relationships rather than to comprehend causal pathways descriptive correlational studies are undertaken. The aim is to describe relationships among variables rather than to infer cause and effect relationships.

Univariate Descriptive Studies

This type of study is conducted to describe the frequency of occurrence of a behavior or condition rather than to study relationships. They do not necessarily focus on only one variable. The primary purpose is to describe the status of each variable and not to relate them to one another.

Two types of descriptive studies from the field of epidemiology are:

(a) Prevalence studies.

(b) Incidence studies.

Prevalence studies: They are done to determine the prevalence rate of some condition at a particular point in time. Findings rely on cross sectional data collected from population at risk. It is like a snapshot of population at risk to determine the extent to which the condition of interest is present.

Formula used is

$$PR = \frac{\text{No. of cases at a given point in time}}{\text{No. in the population at risk of being a case}} \times k$$

k—Number of people for whom the rate is established

Incidence studies: They are used to measure the frequency of developing new cases. It is a longitudinal design for data collection. The researcher must first establish who is at risk for becoming a new case. This means the subject is free of the condition (effect) at the onset of the study.

Formula for IR is

$$IR = \frac{\text{No. of new cases over a given time}}{\begin{array}{c}\text{No. in the population at risk of being a case} \\ \text{(free of effect at the onset)}\end{array}} \times k$$

From the calculations of prevalence and incidence rates, the relative risk is calculated by the formula—

Relative risk is an estimated risk for caseness in one group compared with another.

$$RR = \frac{\text{Rate in one group}}{\text{Rate in another gr.}} \quad (\text{Rate} \geq \text{IR or PR})$$

Strengths of Nonexperimental Research

- Useful because many interesting problems are not amenable to experimentations.
- An efficient means of collecting a large amount of data in relatively short time.
- Strong in realism and hence has an intrinsic appeal for solving practical problems.
- Rarely criticized for artificiality.

Limitations of Nonexperimental Research

- The non-experimental studies are weak in their ability to reveal causal relationship.
- They are susceptible to faulty interpretations.
- Groups are self-selected and not randomized which leads to selection bias.
- Cannot assume that the groups being compared are similar before the occurrence of independent variable.
- Pre-existing differences may contribute to alternative explanations of the outcome.
- In the real world, behaviors, states, attitudes and characteristics are interrelated in complex ways.
- The interpretations are tentative.

CLINICAL TRIALS

Definition: Clinical trials are studies designed to assess clinical intervention's effectiveness for prospective use as a routine intervention for given problem.

In medical and pharmaceutical research, clinical trials adhere to a well-planned sequence of activities.

Phases of Full Clinical Trial

There are four phases of full clinical trial. Full clinical trial is usually conducted to test new drug or an innovative therapy.

Phase I

It starts after initial development of the drug or therapy. It is designed to establish safety and tolerance of the intervention. It aims at determining the optimal dose or strength of the therapy. It involves small scale studies using simple designs. It focuses on developing the best possible and safest treatment.

Phase II

It involves seeking preliminary evidence of the effectiveness of the treatment. Researchers in this phase ascertain the feasibility of launching a more rigorous test. It seeks evidence that the treatment holds promise. It looks for signs of possible side effects of the intervention. It identifies the refinements to improve the intervention.

This phase is considered a pilot test of the treatment. It is designed as a small scale experiment or as a quasi-experiment.

Phase III

In this phase full experimental test of the treatment is done. Randomized clinical trial is conducted. It involves random assignment to an experimental and control group. The RCT is conducted under tightly controlled conditions. It helps to develop evidence about the treatment's efficacy, i.e. new treatment is more efficacious than standard treatment.

It aids in monitoring of adverse effects. It uses a large and heterogeneous sample. Sample is from multiple, geographically dispersed sites. This ensures that findings are not unique to a single setting. In addition, it increases the sample size and the power of the statistical tests.

Multiple site clinical trials are often challenged administratively, require strong oversight, good communication system, staff supervision and data management.

Phase IV

This phase involves studies of the effectiveness of an intervention in the general population. It examines the cost-effectiveness and clinical utility of the new treatment. The focus is on post-approval safety surveillance and long-term consequences over a larger population and time scale.

Drawbacks of Clinical Trials

- Takes many months to recruit and randomize a sufficiently large sample.
- If the population being treated is relatively small, e.g. rare disease, then all the more difficult to generalize the findings and time required may be considerably long.
- It takes years to draw conclusions about the intervention's efficacy.
- One has to wait until all the data have been collected and analyzed.
- Tight control conditions may make them irrelevant for real-life application (artificiality).

SEQUENTIAL CLINICAL TRIAL

Definition: It is an alternative to full clinical trial in which experimental data are continuously analyzed as they become available.

The results accumulate over time and the experiment can be stopped as soon as the evidence is strong enough to support a conclusion about the intervention's efficacy. The sequential clinical trial involves a series of mini-experiments.

Steps of Sequential Clinical Trial (Fig. 5.3)

- The first subject is randomly assigned to either the experimental (E) or control (C) condition.
- The next subject is automatically assigned to the alternative condition.
- This creates a series of randomized paired comparisons.
- Preference is defined on the basis of clinically meaningful outcomes and measured dichotomously, e.g. improved/did not improve.
- Each pair of subjects is compared using preference measures.
- Three possibilities are expected as under – either E is preferred, or C is preferred, and E=C which means two are tied. Such a tied pair is thrown out of the study.

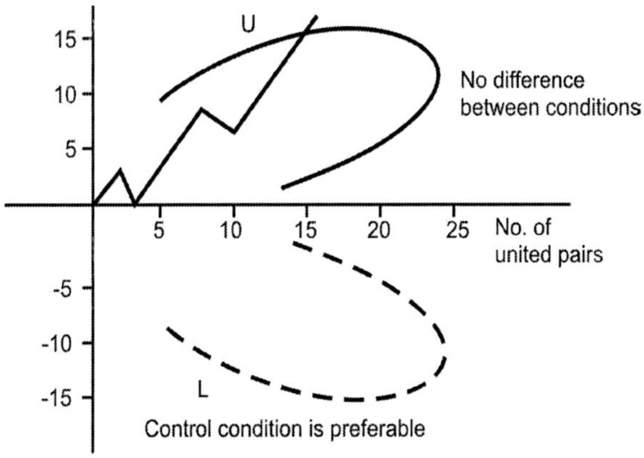

Fig. 5.3: Steps of sequential clinical trial

- All untied paired comparisons are plotted on graphs for which there are pre-established boundaries with decision rules.
- The horizontal axis in the middle of the graph indicates the number of randomized pairs.
- The vertical axis indicates which way the 'preference' comparison turned out.
- The lined butterfly shaped lines designate decision boundaries.
- The procedure of marking preference for each untied pair continues until the plot crosses one of the boundaries (i.e. the line of the butterfly).
- Three stopping rules are as under –
  - When upper boundary (U) is crossed → New treatment is more effective.
  - When lower boundary (L) is crossed → Control conditions are more effective.
  - When middle boundary (M) is crossed → The two treatments are equally effective.

Strengths of Sequential Clinical Trials

- Decisions can be reached much earlier than with traditional designs.
- Applicable in most nursing research.

Limitations

- Not appropriate when three conditions are being compared.
- They are ambiguous when there are many ties.
- They become complicated, if there are multiple outcomes.

PRACTICAL CLINICAL TRIALS

They are also called pragmatic clinical trials. Tunis and others define practical clinical trials as trials for which the hypotheses and study design are formulated based on information needed to make a decision.

- They address practical questions about the benefits and risks of an intervention.
- They consider the cost of the intervention.
- They are sensitive to the issues under scrutiny in effectiveness studies.
- They provide for developing strategies to bridge the gap between efficacy and effectiveness studies.
- They address the issues of utility and practicality of promising interventions much earlier in the evaluation.
- They attempt to achieve methodological purity which may result in clinically meaningless results.
- Efforts to achieve full generalizability may be at risk of losing internal validity and yield unreliable evidence.

Recommendations for Pragmatic Clinical Trials

- Enrollment of diverse study population.
- Recruitment of study participants from a variety of practice settings.
- Longer period of follow-up.
- Inclusion of economic outcomes.
- Comparisons of clinically viable alternatives.
- Use of several research design options, including cluster randomization and delayed treatment designs.
- Hybrid designs that link efficacy and effectiveness research.
- Combination of features of traditional RCTs with elements of effectiveness research.

- Cost-effectiveness of intervention.
- Patient satisfaction
- Minimum restrictions on eligibility for the study.

NURSING INTERVENTION RESEARCH

Definition

These are studies either questioning existing care practices or testing innovations in care that are shaped by nursing values and goals, guided by a strong theoretical basis, informed by recent advances in science and designed to improve the quality of care and health of individuals, families, communities and society.

- They involve an in-depth understanding of the problem and the people for whom the intervention is being developed.
- Careful, collaborative planning with a diverse team.
- Development of an intervention theory to guide the inquiry is must.
- A systematic and progressive sequence that requires a long investment of time to 'get it right' and that places developmental work at a premium.

Phases of Nursing Intervention Research

There are five phases of nursing intervention research. They are:

Phase I: Basic Developmental Phase

During the development phase, researchers address a number of issues relating to both; the design of the intervention and strategies to test it. Conceptualization is a major focus during this phase.

Supported though collaborative discussion, consultations with experts, critical literature reviews and in-depth research to describe and understand the problem. The construct validity is enhanced through efforts to develop an intervention theory. Intervention theory clearly articulates what must be done to achieve desired outcomes.

Interventions theory: It indicates the nature of clinical intervention. It recognizes the factors that would mediate the effects of clinical procedures on expected outcomes. It specifies the clinical inputs. It specifies duration and intensity of the intervention.

Conceptual map is a 'roadmap' for designing and testing the intervention. Developmental work also includes interpersonal relationship cultivation at team level and with variety of stake holders.

The stakeholders are the potential beneficiaries, members of their families, advocates for the target population, community leaders, agents of the intervention, health care administrators and third party payers.

Lack of cooperation, support and trust among key stakeholders is a major pitfall.

To overcome these pitfalls —

- Seek information about the stakeholder's needs and concerns through in-depth research.
- Form an advisory group of key stakeholders.
- Develop channels of communication with stakeholders groups through website etc.

Phase I: Key issues

- Conceptualization of the problems, solutions and strategies.
- Articulation of evidence base for an intervention.
- Identification of potential pitfalls.
- Cultivation of interpersonal relationships.

Phase I: Major Activities

- Concept and theory development.
- Critical synthesis of relevant literature.
- Exploratory and descriptive research.
- Brainstorming with colleagues and team building.
- Consultation with experts.
- Identification of key stakeholders and building partnership with them.

Phase I: Products and Outcomes

- Delineation of an intervention theory.
- Preliminary development of content, intensity, dose and timing of the intervention.
- Development of strategies to overcome pitfalls in implementing and testing the intervention.

- Formulating a design for a pilot study.
- Planning for sponsorship of the pilot study.

Phase II: Pilot Test of the Intervention

- Using simple quasi-experimental designs pilot test of the intervention is done.

Phase II: Key Activities

Pilot test is done:

- To secure preliminary evidence of the intervention's benefits.
- To refine the intervention theory and intervention.
- To finalize intervention protocols.
- To assess the feasibility of a rigorous test.
- It also includes analysis of factors related to recruitment, retention and adherence problems.

Phase III: Full Experimental Test of the Intervention

- Care devoted to wide array of methodologic issues that influence validity and reliability of results.
- Issues related to study and intervention design, sampling, data collection and data analysis are carefully studied and implemented.

Phase IV: Focuses on Effectiveness and the Utility of the intervention in Real world Clinical Settings.

- RE-AIM framework provides for efforts to improve the generalizability of health care research evidence.
- It involves scrutiny of five aspects of a study; namely –
  - Reach— Reaching intended population.
  - Efficacy — Impact on critical outcome.
  - Adoption — Number, proportion and representativeness.
  - Implementation in the form of consistency of delivery of intervention and cost of intervention.
  - Maintenance — of intervention over time, to make it a routine and implementation at institutional level.
- Practical clinical trials that use hybrid designs play an increasingly important role in nursing research.

In research, neither the quantitative nor the qualitative research design is better. Each research approach is useful in different ways and both expand understanding of health care and the nursing profession. The important matter is to choose the methodology that best addresses the questions the researcher is asking and collects the data that are most useful.

More and more nurses are becoming academically astute in the area of research. Unfortunately, education alone does not ensure transfer of what is learned into daily nursing practice. Academic and practice arenas are often, in reality two entirely different cultures. The critical and creative thinking so valued and promoted in the academic environment may fall victim to time and budget constraints within the clinical setting. The implementation of research in practice will depend on inquisitiveness, development of cognitive skills, the ability to question one's own practice, and professional discipline. Nurses must also understand that sometimes research findings may conflict with practices rooted in tradition.

CHAPTER 6

Qualitative Research

Qualitative studies are rooted in research traditions that originated in the disciplines of anthropology, sociology and psychology.

GROUNDED THEORY

Grounded theory has its roots in sociology.

- It seeks to describe and understand the key social psychological and structural processes that occur in a social setting.
- Was developed in 1960s by two sociologists: Glaser and Strauss (1967)
- The focus is on a developing social experience, the social and psychological stages and phases that characterize a particular event or episode.
- The major component is the discovery of a core variable.
- Researches strive to generate comprehensive explanations of phenomena that are grounded in reality.

PHENOMENOLOGY

Phenomenology is a philosophical tradition, developed by Husserl and Heidegger.

- It is concerned with lived experiences of humans.
- It is an approach to thinking about what life experiences of people are like and what they mean.
- It seeks the essence of a phenomenon as experienced by the people under study.
- It also tries to find out the meaning of the phenomenon for those who experience it.

ETHNOGRAPHY

It is the primary research tradition within anthropology, and provides a framework for studying the patterns, life ways and experiences of a cultural group in a holistic fashion.

- In this, researchers engage in extensive fieldwork, often participating to the extent possible in the life of the culture under study.
- Ethnographic research is concerned with broadly defined cultures as well as more narrowly defined cultures.
- The aim of the study is to learn from members of a cultural group, to understand their worldview as they perceive and live it and to describe their customs and norms.

ACTIVITIES IN A QUALITATIVE STUDY

Qualitative research involves cyclic progression of tasks.

- Planning includes steps to be taken to maximize study integrity and implementation involves faithfully following the planned steps.
- The progression of a qualitative study is circular as the researchers are continually examining and interpreting data and making decisions about how to proceed based on what has already been discovered.

Identifying the Research Problem

- Usually begin with a broad topic area.
- The general topic area may be narrowed and clarified on the basis of self-reflection and discussion.

Doing a Literature Review

- Researchers should not consult the literature before collecting data.
- Prior studies might influence conceptualization of the phenomena under study.
- Literature review at the end of the study to obtain a general grounding.
- A relatively small body of relevant previous work at the beginning is appropriate.

Selecting and Gaining Entry into Research Sites

- Identify a site that is consistent.
- Engage in anticipatory fieldwork.
- Identify the most suitable and information—rich environment for the conduct of the study.

- Involvement in negotiations with gatekeepers who have the authority to permit entry into their world.

Developing an Overall Approach

- The research design is an emerging design during the course of data collection.
- Time management for field work.
- Arrange for and test needed equipment, e.g. tape recorders, laptop computers, etc.
- Hiring and training interviewers to assist in the collection of data.
- Securing interpreters and hiring appropriate consultants, transcribers and support staff.

Addressing Ethical Issues

- Develop plans for addressing ethical issues.
- Special concerns in qualitative studies because of the more intimate nature of the relationship that typically develops between researchers and study participants.

Characteristics of a Qualitative Study

- The discussions and observations are loosely structured, allowing for the expression of a full range of beliefs, feelings and behaviors.
- Analysis and interpretation are ongoing, concurrent activities that guide choices about the kinds of people to sample next and the types of questions to ask or observations to make.
- Clustering together related types of narrative information into a coherent scheme.
- Researchers begin to identify themes and categories and use them to build a rich description or theory of the phenomenon.
- Data obtained and the people selected as participants tend to become increasingly focused and purposeful as the conceptualization is developed and refined.
- Concept development and verification shape the sampling process.
- The researcher seeks participants who can confirm and enrich the theoretical understandings and those who can potentially challenge them and lead to further theoretical development.

- Data saturation occurs when themes and categories in the data become repetitive and redundant, such that no new information can be gleaned by further data collection.
- Researchers now take steps to demonstrate the trustworthiness of the data while in the field (Fig. 6.1).

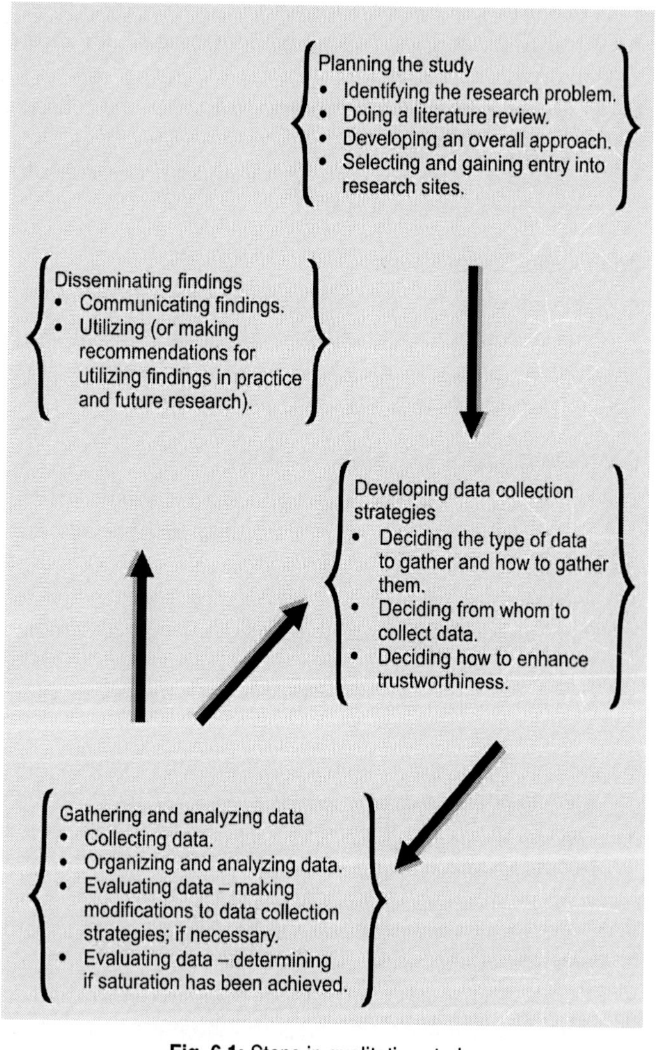

Fig. 6.1: Steps in qualitative study

- Efforts to confirm that the findings accurately reflect the experiences and view points of participants.
- One confirmatory activity involves going back to participants and sharing preliminary interpretations with them so that they can evaluate whether the researchers thematic analysis is consistent with their experiences.
- Development of appropriate strategies for leaving the field.
- Graceful departures and methods of achieving closure are important.

Disseminating Qualitative Findings

- Researchers strive to share their findings with others at conferences and in journal articles.
- The articles should include a summary of prior research in their reports as a means of providing context for the study.
- Qualitative reports are usually filled with rich verbatim passages directly from participants.
- The excepts are used in an evidentiary fashion to support or illustrate researchers' interpretations and thematic construction.
- Qualitative findings often are the basis for formulating hypotheses that are tested by quantitative researchers, for developing measuring instruments for both research and clinical purposes.
- They also contribute for designing effective nursing interventions.
- They help to shape nurse's perceptions of a problem or situation, their conceptualizations of potential solutions and their understanding of patients concerns and experiences.

Qualitative research provides rich information about the psychosocial issues and concerns. It is always been valued by the researchers. Many a times, they have provided grounds for quantitative enquiry.

CHAPTER

7

Quantitative Research

The quantitative research has been popular among researchers for its results being presented in numerical that are easily grasped and less challenged. The objective nature of quantitative study designs have made them more appealing among investigators. The quantitative research has primarily two courses, the experimental and the nonexperimental. This chapter deals with the steps in quantitative research with explanation of researchers activities in each step.

EXPERIMENTAL RESEARCH

- In experimental research, researchers actively introduce an intervention or treatment.
- In medical and epidemiologic research, an experimental study usually is called a controlled trial or clinical trial.
- Experimental studies are explicitly designed to test causal relationship.
- Experimental studies offer the possibility of greater control over extraneous influences.
- Researcher exerts control over independent variables.
- Causal inferences are more plausible.

NONEXPERIMENTAL RESEARCH

- The researchers are bystanders.
- Nonexperimental inquiry is called an observational study.
- Sometimes nonexperimental studies seek to elucidate or detect causal relationships.
- Describe the status and explore existing relationships rather than to test a potential solution to a problem.

STEPS IN A QUANTITATIVE STUDY

- The study moves from research question to obtaining an answer (Fig. 7.1).

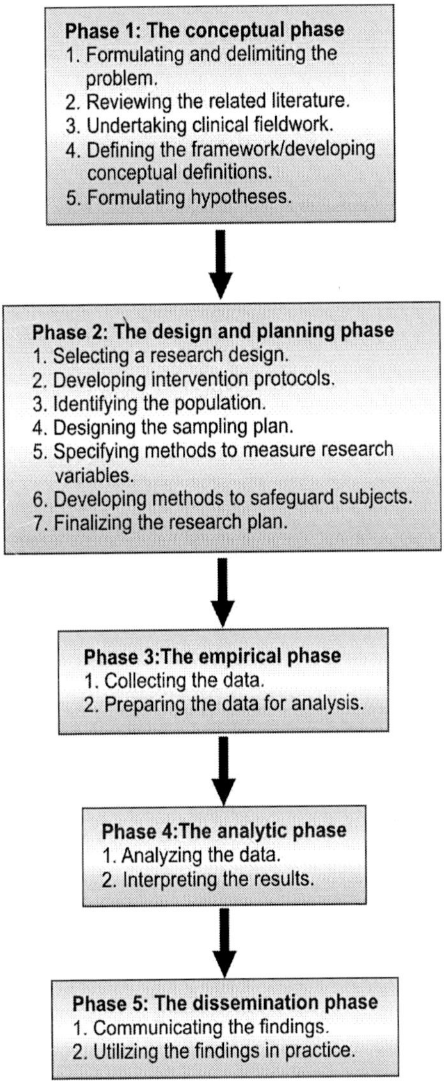

Fig. 7.1: Steps in quantitative study

- The progress of the study is linear sequence of steps.
- Some steps may overlap in certain studies while in certain studies some steps are unnecessary.

Phase I: The Conceptual Phase

- The activities include reading, conceptualizing, theorizing, reconceptualizing and reviewing ideas with colleagues or advisors.
- Researchers call on such skills as creativity, deductive reasoning, insight, and a firm grounding in previous research on the topic of interest.

Step 1: Formulating and Delimiting the Problem

- Identify an interesting, significant research problem and good research questions.
- Researcher must pay close attention to substantive issues, theoretical issues, clinical issues, methodologic issues, and ethic issues.

Step 2: Reviewing the Related Literature

- Quantitative research is conducted within the context of previous knowledge.
- A thorough literature review provides a foundation on which to base new evidence and usually is conducted well before any data are collected.
- Researcher must learn as much as possible about the status of current procedures relating to the topic, to review existing practice guidelines or protocols.

Step 3: Undertaking Clinical Fieldwork

- Spending time in clinical settings, discussing the topic with clinicians and health care administrators, and observing current practices.
- Clinical fieldwork provides perspectives on recent clinical trends, current diagnostic procedures, and relevant health care delivery models.
- This fieldwork helps the researchers better understand affected clients and the settings in which care is provided.
- It is valuable in developing methodologic strategies for strengthening the study.

- Discover the need for research assistants, or bilingual interpreters.

Step 4: Defining the Framework and Developing Conceptual Definitions

- Research in the context of a theoretical framework, the findings may have broader significance and utility.
- A conceptual rationale and a clear sense of the concepts under study.
- Important task of development of conceptual definitions.

Step 5: Formulating Hypothesis

- A hypothesis is a statement of the researcher's expectations about relationships between study variables.
- Hypotheses are predictions of expected outcomes.
- Hypothesis state the relationships researchers expect to find as a result of the study.
- Research question asks how the concepts are related and hypothesis predicts the answer.
- Quantitative designs test hypothesis through statistical analysis.

Phase II: The Design and Planning Phase

- Decisions about the methods and procedures to be used to address the research question and plan for actual collection of data marks the 2nd phase.
- Researchers have considerable flexibility and must make many decisions.

Step 6: Selecting of Research Design

- The research design is the overall plan for obtaining answers to the questions being studied and for handling some of the difficulties encountered during the research process.
- Researchers specify which specific design will be adopted and what will be done to minimize bias and enhance the interpretability of results.
- The design tends to be highly structured and controlled. Decisions about how often data will be collected, what types

of comparisons will be made and where the study will take place; are made.

- The research design is the architectural backbone of the study.

Step 7: Developing protocols for the Interventions

- Participants are exposed to different treatment or conditions.
- Intervention protocol for the study is developed.
- What the biofeedback of treatment would entail.
- How long the treatment would last.
- What the alternative condition would be.
- The goal is to have all subjects in each group treated in the same way (This step is not necessary in nonexperimental research).

Step 8: Identifying the Population

- To know what characteristics the study participants should possess and to whom study results can be generalized.
- Must identify the population to be studied.
- A population is all the individuals or objects with common, defining characteristics.

Step 9: Designing the Sampling Plan

- Collect data from a sample, which is a subset of the population.
- Use of samples is more practical and less costly than collecting data from entire population.
- But the sample might not adequately reflect the population's traits. Hence, assess the samples adequacy for representativeness.
- The sampling plan specifies in advance how the sample will be selected and recruited, and how many subjects there will be.

Step 10: Specifying Methods to Measure the Research Variables

- Must develop or borrow methods to measure the research variables as accurately as possible.
- Quantitative data collection approaches include: self reports, observations, biophysiologic measurements.
- The task of measuring research variables and developing a data collection plan is a complex and challenging process.

Step 11: Developing Methods to Safeguard Human or Animal Rights

- Need to develop procedures to ensure that the study adheres to ethical principles.
- Need to determine whether the rights of the participants and subjects have been adequately protected.
- To present to external review committee or institutional ethical board.

Step 12: Reviewing and Finalizing the Research Plan

- Evaluate the readability of any written material.
- Pretest measuring instruments to assess its adequacy.
- Have research plan critiqued by peers, consultants or other reviewers.
- Submit the research proposal for financial assistance to appropriate authorities.
- Inculcate the suggested improvements.

Phase III : The Empirical Phase

This phase involves collecting research data and preparing it / them for analysis. Most time-consuming part of the research.

Step 13: Collection of Data

- The actual collection of data as per pre-established plan.

Step 14: Preparing the Data for Analysis

- Coding is the process of translating verbal data into numeric form.
- Transferring the data from written documents on computer files for subsequent analysis.

Phase IV: The Analytic Phase

- Quantitative data is subjected to analysis and interpretation.

Step 15: Analyzing the Data

- Process and analyze data in orderly, coherent fashion.
- Statistical procedures are applied.
- Statistical analyses cover a broad range of techniques, from simple to complex and sophisticated methods.
- It helps to grasp the key concepts easily.

Step 16 : Interpreting the Results

- Interpretation is the process of making sense of study results and examining their implications.
- Explain the findings in light of prior evidence, theory and researcher's own clinical experience.
- Explain the adequacy of methods used in the study.
- Determine clinical implications of the findings.
- Suggest if further research is required before utilization of findings can be recommended.

Phase V: The Dissemination Phase

- The study results need to be disseminated to complete the researcher's responsibilities in a given study.

Step 17 : Communicating the Findings

- Final task of research project is to prepare research report.
- RR can be shared with others.
- Can be in the form of term papers, dissertations, journal articles, presentations at conferences, etc.
- Thus, they are made available to broad, international audience.

Step 18 : Utilizing Findings in Practice

- Ideally, it is the concluding step of high-quality study.
- Use of findings in practice settings need to be planned carefully.
- Recommendations are to be made in RR about how the evidence from the study could be incorporated into the practice of nursing.
- Identify opportunities to disseminate the findings to practicing nurses.

A recommendation for replication of the study, multiple uses of the instrument, etc. may be made in the research report.

Thus quantitative research collects numerical data/quantified data, uses scientific method of problem solving and provides with the solutions scientifically tested and statistically analyzed.

CHAPTER 8

Noninterventional Research Designs

These research designs do not involve intervention. They are popular study designs. These are used for conducting study for a specific purpose. A very small sample of experts may be used as in Delphi studies on one hand and a very large sample may be recruited as in surveys on the other hand. These studies are applicable in a restricted area of practice and may yield very strong evidence. Many a times, they form the basis for interventional studies.

TYPES OF NONINTERVENTIONAL RESEARCH

Outcome Research

It is conducted to document the effectiveness of health care services. They play an important role in policy research. The design overlaps to some degree with evaluation research. But it is a more global assessment of nursing and health care services. The input data for outcome research comes from quality assessment and quality assurance functions.

It represents a response to increased demands from policy makers, insurers and public. It is in terms of both improved patient outcomes and costs. Outcome research provides for appraisal of the quality of nursing care— as distinct from the care provided by overall health care system.

It aids in linking patient outcomes to specific nursing actions or interventions, distinct from the actions of other members of the health care team. Health care is influenced by factors outside the health care delivery system hence it is difficult to attribute the outcome to only nursing interventions. Variety of designs, are used for study and sampling strategies, data collection and analysis approaches. Complex multidisciplinary nature of outcomes research provides for methodologic creativity.

Survey Research

A survey is designed to obtain information about the prevalence, distribution and interrelations of variables within a population, e.g. decennial census

When surveys use samples of individuals, they may be referred to as sample surveys.

Information obtained by self-report from study participants. Study participants respond to a series of questions posed by the investigator.

Merits of Survey Research

- Survey research yield large quantity of data.
- The data are quantitative.
- The survey data can be cross-sectional or longitudinal.
- The research flexibility and broadness of scope.
- They can be applied to many populations.
- They focus on a wide range of topics.
- Information can be used for many purposes.

Demerits of Survey Research

- Information is usually relatively superficial.
- Information is rarely about the complexities of human behavior and feelings.
- Better suited for extensive rather than intensive analysis.
- Only available respondents provide the information.
- Non experimental study and inherent drawbacks of the observational study.
- Limited to willing and eligible respondents.
- Information by direct questioning only, can be obtained.
- Include questions that mostly require brief responses.

Methods of Collecting Survey Data

- Personal interviews
- Telephone interviews
- Questionnaires
- Audio-CASI (Computer Assisted Self Interview)

Personal Interview

- Most respected method.
- Also called face-to-face interviews.
- Costly in terms of personnel and time.
- Best method of collecting survey data.
- Quality and accuracy of information is good.
- Refusal rate is low.

Telephone Interview

- Less costly.
- Interviewer is unknown.
- Respondents may be uncooperative.
- Convenient when interview is short, specific, not too personal.
- May be difficult for certain groups of respondents including low income groups who do not have telephone, elderly and those with hearing impaired.

Mixed Mode Strategy

In this, the interviewer first attempts to interview a sample member by telephone. If initial attempts fail, then attempts a personal interview or goes to the respondents home with a cellular phone and personally asks the respondent to complete the interview by phone.

Questionnaires

They are self-administered. They are also called (Self Administered Questionnaires) (SAQs). Respondents read questions on a written form and give their answers in writing. Respondents differ in their reading levels. Respondents differ in their communication in writing. Questions must be worded clearly and simply. SAQs are economical. They are not appropriate for certain type of population e.g. children, elderly, etc.

Computer Assisted Self Interview

It is a state of the art approach for giving respondents more privacy. It is useful for population with literacy problems. Respondents sit at a computer and listen to question over headphones. Respondents enter their responses directly onto the keyboard without the interviewer having to see the responses.

Delphi Surveys

These are developed as a tool for short-term forecasting. The telephone involves a panel of experts who are asked to complete several rounds of questionnaires focusing on their judgements about a topic of interest.

Merits of Delphi Research

- Multiple interactions with participant experts.
- No face to face discussions.
- Responses to each round of questionnaires are analyzed, summarized and returned to experts with new questionnaires.
- The experts then reformulate their opinions with the panel's viewpoint in mind.
- The procedure is usually repeated at least three times until a general consensus is obtained.
- Efficient means of combining the experts of geographically dispersed group.
- Experts are spared of formal meeting thus saving their time and expenses.
- A persuasive or prestigious expert cannot have an undue influence on the opinions of others.
- All the panel members are on equal footing.
- Anonymity encourages greater candor.
- Useful methodologic tool for problem solving, planning and forecasting.

Demerits of Delphi Research

- Time consuming for the researcher.
- Experts need to be solicited.
- Questionnaires to be prepared and mailed.
- Responses to be analyzed.
- Results are to be summarized.
- New questionnaires to be prepared.
- Cooperation may fade in later rounds.
- Attrition is possible.
- Concern about how to define consensus.

In addition to these several study, designs are adopted for a specific purpose of the study. These include secondary analysis, replication studies, methodologic research, evaluation studies, etc.

Triangulation of different types of data, and use of mixed method design are the two major strengths of these studies. While critiquing these studies, the advantages of both of the abovementioned should be weighed.

CHAPTER 9

Sampling

Sampling is a part of everyday life. Quantitative and qualitative researchers have different approaches to sampling. Quantitative researchers seek to select samples that allow to achieve statistical conclusion validity and to generalize their results. A sampling plan is developed specifying how to select study participants and how many to select in a particular study. Sampling is an important aspect of feasibility of a study. Sampling is responsible for the strength of the findings in a study.

Qualitative researchers go for holistic approach. Sampling decisions during the course of data collection mark the qualitative studies. These decisions are based on the informational needs and theoretical needs of the study.

DEFINITIONS

Sampling: Sampling is a process of selecting a portion of the population to represent the entire population so that inferences about the population can be made.

Population: It is the entire aggregation of cases in which a researcher is interested.

Population is not restricted to human subjects, e.g. blood samples, hospital record files, schools, etc. are all population.

Target population: It is the aggregate of cases about which the researcher would like to generalize.

Accessible population: It is also called source population. It is the aggregate of cases that conform to designated criteria and that are accessible as subjects for a study.

Sample: It is a subset of population element who would actually be recruited for the study and who would participate in the study. This group meets the eligibility criteria of the population under study.

An element: It is the most basic unit about which information is collected.

A representative sample: It is the sample whose key characteristics closely approximate those of the population. If the sample is not representative then the external validity and the construct validity of the study is at risk.

Eligibility criteria: Researchers must specify criteria that define who is included in the population. The exact criteria by which it would be decided whether an individual would or would not be classified as a member of study population are called eligibility criteria.

- They are also called inclusion criteria.
- Sometimes a population is defined in terms of characteristics that people must not possess. They are called exclusion criteria.
- The sample should be representative of the population construct in which researcher is interested.
- The construct validity of the study is enhanced when there is a good match between the eligibility criteria and the population construct.

Eligibility criteria may reflect on (a) cost constraints, e.g. translators' charges, (b) practical constraints, e.g. having impaired population, (c) people's ability to participate in a study, e.g. mentally ill clients, (d) design considerations, e.g. internal validity of the study as it controls extraneous variables.

SAMPLING TECHNIQUES

There are two sampling techniques. They are—

(a) Non-probability sampling (Fig. 9.1).
(b) Probability Sampling.

TYPES OF NON-PROBABILITY SAMPLING

Convenience Sampling

- Entails using the most conveniently available people as study participants.
- Also called accidental sample.
- Available subjects might be atypical of population of interest with regard to critical variables.
- Subjects may be unknown to the researcher.

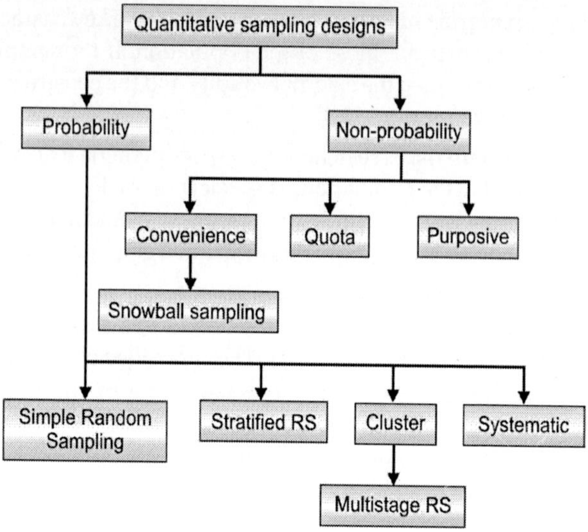

Fig. 9.1: Quantitative sampling design

- Technique used: Stopping signal at a street corner, Volunteers to notices or press advertisements, chat room messages on internet.

Snowball Sampling

- Also called network sampling or chain sampling.
- Variant of convenience sampling.
- Early sample members (called seeds) are asked to refer other people who meet the eligibility criteria.
- Useful for population with variables under study are difficult to identify (people who are afraid of hospital, people with rare disease, etc.)
- Mostly used by qualitative researchers.
- Convenience sampling is the weakest form of sampling.

Quota Sampling

A quota sample is one in which the researcher identifies population strata and determines how many participants are needed from each stratum.

- Researcher must know population characteristics.

- Diverse segments of population characteristics are to be represented in the sample.
- The proportion of population characteristics should be preferably same as in the population.
- The strata are based on gender, income, education, etc.
- The quota sample must include selection of study participants so that the sample contains the correct number of cases from each stratum.
- Quota sample reflects the viewpoint of the population.
- Does not require sophisticated skills or a lot of effort.
- Surprisingly not popular among researchers.
- Stratification should be based on one or more variables that would reflect important differences in the dependent variable under study.
- Quota sampling is similar to convenience sampling procedurally except for identifying the strata and desired representation for each of the strata.
- Shares weaknesses same as convenience sampling.

Purposive Sampling

- Also called judgmental sampling.
- Researcher's knowledge about the population can be used to hand-pick sample members.
- Researcher purposefully decides to select subjects.
- Subjects knowledgeable about the issues under study are selected typically.
- Sampling is subjective.
- No external, objective method for assessing the typicalness of the selected subjects.
- Newly developed instruments can be effectively pretested and evaluated with purposive sampling of diverse type of people.
- Purposive sampling used when researchers want a sample of experts, e.g. Delphi studies.
- Frequently used by qualitative researchers.

Evaluation of Non-probability Sampling

- Rarely representative of the population.
- Some segments of the study variables may be under represented.

- Sampling bias is inherent which may have the results that are misleading.
- Very convenient.
- Economical.
- Does not require any special skill or resources.
- Careful selection of sample, conservative interpretation of results and replication of study with new samples, yield substantive results that can be trusted and used.

Measures to Enhance the Representativeness

- Identify the extraneous variables of importance.
- Try to eliminate the variable from extraneous variables as far as possible.
- Make the heterogeneous popular in more homogeneous.

PROBABILITY SAMPLING

- Involves random selection of elements from a population.
  Random sampling involves a selection process in which each element in the population has an equal and independent chance of being selected.
- It is a complex and technical topic.

Types of Probability Sampling

Simple Random Sampling

- Most basic probability sampling design.
- Researcher establishes a sampling frame, i.e. the list of the elements from which the sample will be chosen.
- A population may be defined in terms of an existing sampling frame.
- Then the elements are numbered.
- A table of random numbers is then used to draw a sample of desired size.
- A sample selected randomly is not subject to researcher's biases.
- Randomly selected sample may or may not be representative.
- The random selection ensures that the differences in the attributes of the sample and the population are purely a function of chance.

- It is a laborious and time consuming process, particularly if the population is large.
- Relatively inefficient procedure.
- It is not always possible to get a listing of every element in the population.
- Tossing a coin, lottery method are methods of simple random sampling.

Stratified Random Sampling

- In stratified random sampling, the population is first divided into two or more strata.
- The aim is to enhance representativeness.
- Stratified sampling designs subdivide the population into homogeneous subsets from which an appropriate number of elements are selected at random.
- Stratification is usually based on demographic variables such as age, gender, etc.
- Stratifying attributes must be known in advance.
- Information about stratifying variables may not be available.
- Random sampling with stratification needs information about a person's status in a stratum before random selection unlike quota sampling, where researcher can ask prospective subjects questions that determine their eligibility for a particular stratum.
- Stratified sampling can guarantee the appropriate representation of different segments of the population.
- Stratifying variables divide the population into unequal sub-populations.
- The researcher might select subjects in proportion to the size of the stratum in the population using proportionate stratified sampling.
- When researchers are interested in understanding differences among strata, proportionate sampling may result in insufficient numbers for making comparisons.
- Disproportionate sampling design is suited when comparisons are sought between strata of greatly unequal size.
- With disproportionate sampling, it is necessary to make an adjustment to the data to arrive at the best estimate of overall population values.

- This adjustment process is known as weighting and is a simple mathematic computation.
- Stratified random sampling sharpens the precision and representativeness of the final sample.
- It provides a means of including a sufficient number of cases in the sample by over sampling for that stratum.
- Cannot be used, if information on the critical variables is unavailable.
- Requires more labor and effort than SRS.

Cluster Sampling

- For large population, it is impossible to get a listing of all elements.
- Large scale surveys never use simple or stratified random sampling.
- In cluster sampling, there is a successive random sampling of units.
- The first unit is large grouping called clusters.
- A random sampling of clusters.
- A random sampling of elements from these each of the clusters.
- The usual procedure for selecting samples from a general population is to sample successively such administrative units as states, census tracts and then households.
- This approach is also called multistage sampling because of the successive stages in cluster sampling.
- The clusters can be selected either by simple or stratified methods.
- The final selection from within a cluster may also be performed by simple or stratified random sampling.
- Less accurate than simple or stratified random sampling.
- More economical and practical when the population is large and widely dispersed.

Systematic Sampling

- Involves the selection of every 'k'th case from a list, such as every 10th person on a patient list or 100th person, etc.
- The population is not narrowly defined. It is similar to convenient sampling.

- Systematic sampling is essentially random sampling.
- The desired sample size of the population is established at some number (n). the size of the population is N. Sample interval is estimated by formula K = N/n.
- Every 'K'th element on the list is sampled.
- It is less laborious and hence popular.
- Same results as those of SRS in a more efficient manner.
- Can be used for stratified lists.

Evaluation of Probability Sampling

- Only viable method of obtaining representative samples.
- Allows researchers to estimate the magnitude of sampling error.
- Permits estimates of the degree of error.
- Drawback of inconvenience and complexity.
- May be beyond the scope of the researcher unless the population is narrowly defined.
- Preferred and most respected method of obtaining sample elements.
- Often impractical.
- The quality of the sampling plan is of particular importance in survey research because purpose of surveys is to obtain descriptive information about the prevalence of average values for a population.
- All surveys use probability samples usually cluster samples.
- Probability samples are rarely used in experimental and quasi-experimental studies because the main focus of such inquiries is on between – group differences rather than absolute values for a population.

Implementing a Sampling Plan in Quantitative Studies

- Decisions are made about the sampling design and sample size.

Steps in Sampling

1. Identifying the population— Begin with a clear idea about the target population to which the results of the study would be generalized.

2. Specify the eligibility criteria— The eligibility criteria should be as specific as possible. Both inclusion and exclusion criteria are specified.
3. Specify the sampling plan— It includes:
   - The method of drawing a sample
   - How large the sample will be.

     Perform power analysis if you can to determine the desired number of subjects.

     As large a sample as possible and as representative a sample as possible should be recruited.
4. Recruit the sample— Recruit the subjects as per plan.
   - Take prior permission of institutions.
   - Take informed consent.
   - Seek necessary cooperation.

Points to be Considered while Recruiting the Sample

- Identify the eligible candidates.
- Persuade them to participate in the study.
- Early planning and field work for deciding the best source for recruiting potential participants.
- Administrative approval is a must.
- One site or multisite sample collection.
- Screening the instrument development.
- Actually gaining cooperation of study participants.
- Recruitment method à face to face recruitment is more effective.
- Courtesy—Recruiters to be pleasant, courteous, non-threatening and preferably of same gender, race and ethnicity as of the study participant.
- Persistence—May be required sometimes.
- Incentives—Gifts and monetary incentives to increase participation.
- Research Benefits—To the individual and to the society must be carefully explained.
- Sharing Results— People are at times interested to know the results of their contribution to the study.
- Convenience—Collect data at a time and location that is convenient for participants. Arrange for transportation or care of their young children need to be thought about.

- Endorsement—Study to be endorsed/acknowledged by a person or organization that has prospective subjects confidence and to communicate this to them.
  - Institution serving as a research setting.
  - Funding agency.
  - Respected community group/person.
  - Press releases in advance.
- Assurance— Who will see the data and how it will be used, how confidentiality will be maintained must be told to the subjects.

SAMPLING IN QUALITATIVE RESEARCH

- Mostly use small, non-probability random samples.
- Concerned with measuring attributes and relationships in a population.
- A representative sample is needed to ensure that the measurements accurately reflect and can be generalized.
- Aim is to discover meaning and to uncover multiple realities.
- Generalizability is not a guiding consideration.
- Individuals are not always the units of analysis in qualitative research.
- Incidents or experiences are often the basis of analysis.
- Small number of informants can generate a large sample of analysis.
- No rules for sample size.
- A random sample is not the best method of selecting people who will make good informants.
- Good informants— People who are knowledgeable, articulate, reflective and willing to talk at length with researchers.
- Hence, non-probability sampling is best suited.

Types of Qualitative Sampling

- Convenience sampling
- Snowball sampling
- Purposive sampling
  - Maximum variation sampling
  - Homogeneous sampling

- Extreme (deviant) case sampling.
- Intensity sampling
- Typical case sampling
- Critical case sampling
- Criterion sampling
- Theory-based sampling
- Sampling confirming and disconfirming cases.

- Theoretical sampling in grounded theory.
- Sampling in ethnography
- Sampling in phenomenological studies
- Sampling in grounded theory studies.

Convenience Sampling

- Also called volunteer sample.
- Used when researchers want to have potential participants come forward and identify themselves.
- Emphasis is on obtaining a diverse rather than representative sample.
- It is easy and efficient but not much preferred.
- In qualitative studies, the main emphasis is on to extract the greatest possible information from the few cases in the sample.
- Convenience sample may not provide the most information rich sources.
- It is economical and easy way to begin the sampling process.

Snowball Sampling

- Ask early informants to make referrals to other study participants.
- More cost-efficient and practical.
- Less time required to screen people to determine whether they are appropriate for study.
- With an introducer as a referring person, researchers may have an easier time establishing a trusting relationship with new participants.
- Researchers can specify the characteristics of their new participants more readily.

- Referrals to people who would add other dimensions to the sample, i.e. variations in age, race, socioeconomic status, etc.
- Weakness— The eventual sample might be restricted to a small network of acquaintances.
- Quality of the referrals may be affected by whether the referring sample member trusted the researcher and truly wanted to cooperate.

Purposive Sampling

Qualitative sampling may begin with volunteers informants and may be supplemented with new participants through snowballing.

- Eventually sampling evolves to be a purposive sampling strategy.
- It means selecting cases that will most benefit study.
- A diverse strategies of purposive sampling are used by qualitative researchers.
- Carefully choose particular exemplars in order to enhance the researchers' understanding of the phenomena.

  Maximum variation sampling: Involves purposefully selecting cases with a wide range of variation on dimensions of interest.
  - Researchers invite challenges to emerging conceptualizations.
  - Involves ensuring of people with diverse backgrounds represented in the sample.
  - Involves deliberate attempts to include people with different viewpoints about the phenomenon under study.

  Homogeneous sampling: Deliberately reduces variation and permits a more focused inquiry.
  - To understand a particular group of people especially well.
  - It is used to select people for group interviews.

  Extreme (deviant) case sampling: Provides opportunities for learning from the most unusual and extreme informants (i.e. outstanding successes and extreme failures).
  - Extreme cases are rich in information because they are special in some way.
  - Sometimes, extreme case can distort understanding of a phenomenon.

Intensity sampling: Similar to extreme case but has less emphasis on the extremes.

- Involve information rich cases that manifest the phenomenon of interest intensely.
- The goal is to select rich cases that offer strong example of the phenomenon.

Typical case sampling: Involves the selection of participants who illustrate or highlight what is typical or average.

- The resulting information creates a qualitative profile illustrating typical manifestations of the phenomenon being studied.

Critical case sampling: Involves selecting important cases regarding the phenomenon of interest.

- Look for the particularly good story that illuminates critical aspects of the phenomenon.

Criterion sampling: Involves studying cases that meet a predetermined criterion of importance.

- It is used in mixed method studies.
- To select cases meeting certain criteria for in depth study.

Theory-based sampling: Involves the selection of people or incidents on the basis of their potential representation of important theoretical constructs.

- Based on a prior theory which is being examined qualitatively.

Sampling confirming and disconfirming cases:

- Often used towards end of qualitative data collection.
- Researcher notes trends and patterns in the data.
- Emerging conceptualizations need to be checked.
- Confirming cases are additional cases that fit researchers' conceptualizations and offer enhanced credibility.
- Disconfirming cases do not fit and serve to challenge researchers' interpretations.
- These negative cases may offer new insights about how the original conceptualization needs to be revised or expanded.

Regarding Sampling the Researcher's Must Know:

- The setting in which the study is taking place.
- The goal to be actively and purposefully pursue the best.
- To start with excellent examples of the phenomenon being studied.

Theoretical Sampling

- Method of sampling used in grounded theory.
- Glaser defined, "The process of data collection for generating theory whereby the analyst jointly collects, codes and analyzes his data and decides what data to collect next and where to find them, in order to develop his theory as it emerges."
- Guided by the developing grounded theory.
- It is not single, unidirectional.
- It is a complex technique and requires researchers to be involved with multiple lines and directions as they go back and forth between data and categories.
- Purpose is to discover categories and their properties.
- To offer inter relationships that occur in substantive theory.
- Whom to ask next? is the basic question.
- Sample groups are not chosen before the research begins.
- Involves more than selecting informants.
- Observation and other means of data collection play a big role in helping researchers understand a culture.

Sampling in Ethnography

- Initially the approach is 'big-net'—Mingling with and having conversations with as many members of the culture under study as possible.
- Rely on small number of key informants who are:
  - Highly knowledgeable about the culture.
  - Develop on going relationships with researcher.
  - The main link to the inside.
- Key informants chosen purposively.
- Guided by the ethnographers informed judgements.
- Depends on ethnographers' prior knowledge to construct a relevant framework.

- Different types of key informants based on roles or other distinctive characteristics.
- For final selection, participants'
  - Level of knowledge about the culture.
  - Willingness to collaborate, are the criteria.
- Involves more than selecting informants.
- Observations and other means of data collection play a big role in helping researchers understand a culture.
- 'Whom to sample' and 'what to sample' decisions are very important.
- Decisions about observing events and activities about examining records and artifacts and about exploring places that provide clues about the culture.

Sampling in Phenomenological Studies

- Tend to rely on very small samples of participants (10 or fewer)
- *Guiding principle:* All participants must have experienced the phenomenon and must be able to articulate what it is like to have lived that experience.
- Use of criterion sampling method.
- The criterion is the experience with the phenomenon under study.
- To explore diversity of individual experiences.
- Look for people with demographic or other differences who have shared a common experience.

Sampling in Grounded Theory Studies

- Samples of about 20 to 30 people.
- Use theoretical sampling.
- The goal is to select informants who can best contribute to the evolving theory.
- Sampling, data collection, data analysis and theory construction occur concurrently.
- So, study participants are selected serially and contingently.
- Sampling evolves as —
  - Begins with a general notion of where and with whom to start.

- First few cases solicited purposively by convenience or snowball sampling.
- Early part of the study may have maximum variation sampling to gain insights into the range and complexity of the phenomenon under study.
- Sample adjusted in an ongoing fashion.
- Sampling continues until saturation is achieved.
- Final sampling often includes a search for confirming and disconfirming cases to test, refine, and strengthen the theory.

Critiquing Sampling Plans

- Important is to avoid sampling bias.
- Study the plans for:
  - The type of sampling approach used.
  - The population under study.
  - The eligibility criteria – Inclusion and exclusion
  - The nature of the setting.
  - The nature of study groups.
  - The number of participants in the study.
  - The rationale for the sample size.
  - The description of the main characteristics of participants.
  - The number and characteristics of potential subjects who declined to participate in the study.
- Whether the researcher made good sampling decisions in case the sample is inadequate.

Critiquing Quantitative Sampling Plans

- The sampling plan affects the study's validity— the internal validity, the construct validity, the external validity and the statistical conclusion validity are influenced.
- If sample is small – statistical conclusion validity is likely to be undermined.
- Restrictive inclusion/eligibility criteria – enhance benefits of internal validity. But is detrimental to construct validity and external validity.
- Sample may not be representative if sampling strategy is weak or sample size is small.

- In cases of risk for bias, steps to estimate the direction and degree of bias must be taken.
- If certain segments of population refuse to participate, then a biased sample can result.
- The research report should provide information about response rates and about possible non response bias.
- Study for attrition bias.
- If the target population is defined broadly, researchers may have missed opportunities to control extraneous variables and the gap between the accessible and target population may be too great.
- Draw conclusions about reasonableness of generalizing the findings from the researcher's sample to accessible population and from accessible population to a broader target population.
- If sampling plan is seriously flawed, generalizing findings is risky.
- Replication of study with another sample is advocated.

Critiquing Qualitative Sampling Plan

- Evaluate sampling plan in terms of its adequacy and appropriateness.
- Adequacy in terms of sample size, information.
- Results are richly textured and complete.
- Appropriateness — Participants who supply best information.
- Use of strategy that yields the fullest possible understanding of the phenomenon of interest.
- The potential for transferability of the findings to be judged.
- Fittingness is the degree of congruence between original study sample and the people at another site to which the finding might be applied.
- Thick description of the sample.
- The context in which the study was carried out.

The sampling technique and implementation of sampling plan are important in a study for its strength and generalizability.

CHAPTER

10

Pilot Study and Data Collection

In a study, high-quality data collection methods are must for the accuracy and robustness of conclusions. In developing a data collection plan, researchers must think of the kind of evidence they want to provide for nursing practice through their study. Some amount of data may already exist. The researcher must be in a position to judge its relevance and applicability in their study.

TYPES OF DATA

1. Unstructured data.
2. Structured data.

Unstructured Data Collection

Qualitative self-report techniques: These include unstructured interviews, semi-structured interviews, focus group interviews, joint interviews, life histories, oral histories, critical incidents, diaries and journals, the think aloud method, photo elicitation interviews and self report narratives on internet.

Unstructured observational methods: These include participant observation, recording observations, descriptive observations, focused observations, selective observations; all of which may be single positioning, multiple positioning or mobile positioning. Descriptive field notes, reflective filed notes, methodologic field notes, theoretical notes and personal notes are other methods of unstructured observations.

Structured Data Collection

Structured self report: Instruments include open ended questions, closed ended questions which may be dichotomous questions or multiple choice questions, cafeteria questions, rank order questions, forced choice questions, rating scales, checklists and visual analogue scales.

Composite scales: For example, Likert scales by psychologist Rensis Likert; which is a five point rating scale. Several declarative items on a topic are presented and the respondents express their viewpoint by rating the items. 10 or more items in a scale. The items are worded positively and negatively intermittently or alternatively to avoid tend bias. Requires skill and hard work to construct.

Semantic differential scales: For measuring psychological traits. They are flexible, and easy to construct.

Cognitive and neuropsychological tests: For example I.Q. tests, Mini Mental state examination, Q Sorts which include reaction to phrases on cards and vignettes which have reaction to brief descriptions of situations.

Structured interviews

Structured observations

Biophysiologic measures.

Purposes of Biophysiologic Measures

- In studies, basic biophysiologic processes have relevance to nursing care.
- To describe the physiologic outcomes of nursing and health care.
- To evaluate a specific nursing interventions.
- To assess product.
- To evaluate the measurement and recording of biophysiologic information gathered by nurses.
- To collect data in studies of the correlates of physiologic functioning, in patients with health problems.

PILOT STUDY

Definition: The pilot study is a small preliminary investigation of the same general character as the major study, which is designed to acquaint the researcher with problems that can be corrected in preparation for the large research projects.

Characteristics

- Should have the objects 10 percent of the anticipated sample size considered for main study.

- It is a small scale study dress rehearsal.
- Includes subjects other than those who will participate in actual study.
- It tests the data collection instrument.
- The site of data collection should preferably be other than the site selected for main study.

Objectives

- To test as many elements of the research proposal as possible.
- To provide for correction of any element that does not work as intended.
- To foresee the problems of sampling and data collection that can be remedied.
- To identify the weaknesses in the study design that may pose threat to internal and external validity of the study.
- To determine the cost of the study and test its cost-effectiveness.
- To maintain the confidentiality of the study subjects and data collected.
- To determine the time and pit falls and errors that may prove costly and inappropriate for the study that may be identified and avoided.
- To seek sponsors for the actual study.
- To make improvements in the research project.
- To detect problems that must be eradicated before the major study is attempted.

Every research study serves as a pilot study for the anticipatory large study.

Significance/Advantages of Pilot Study

- It tells us about the completeness, accuracy and convenience of sampling frame from which it is proposed to select the sample.
- It unfolds the variability within the population to be surveyed. It is important for determining the sample size.
- It helps in bringing out the inadequacies of the draft questionnaire.
- Throws light on several difficulties in the study.

- Shows the effectiveness of the training of the personnel for collecting data.
- Allays interviewer's fear about overtly sensitive questions and builds their self confidence.
- Tests interviewer's stamina to work under conditions of personal discomfort, stress and fatigue.
- Tests the efficiency of the survey organization in the field.
- Helps in identifying the needs for different kinds of equipment, vehicles necessary during the project.
- Provides data for making estimates of time and costs for completing various phases of the project and shows ways to effect savings.
- Scale of pilot study will depend on the availability of resources like time, money and personnel.
- Provides for initial analysis of the adequacy of the questionnaire and the training instructions and supervision under field conditions.
- Aids to identify parts of the instrument package that are difficult for pretest subjects.
- Helps to identify objectionable or offensive questions.
- Assesses the sequencing of instrument to be sensible.
- Determines the needs for training of data collection staff.
- Determines whether the measurement yields data with sufficient variability.

Data Collection Plan

Step 1: Determine the nature of data required.
  - Are the data needs extensive?
  - Prioritize the list of needs.

Step 2: Determine the tools to be used.
  - Are the tools available— seek permission
  - Self prepared tools — get validated.
  - Unable to prepare tools— change the hypothesis.
  - Modify the available tool if required.

Step 3: Arrange measures in an appropriate sequence.

Step 4: Pretest entire instrument package.

Step 5: Make necessary revisions to instruments.

Step 6: Develop data collection forms and protocols;

Develop data management procedures.

- Time of data collection.
- Duration.
- Personnel to be used and trained.
- Permission from gatekeepers of the area.
- Location of data collection.
- Confidentiality and ethical issues.

Step 7: Collect the data.

Step 8: Manage data according to data management plan.

Determinants of Data Requirement

- Testing the hypothesis.
- Sample characteristics description.
- Controlling extraneous variables.
- Analyzing potential biases.
- Understanding subgroup effects.
- Interpreting results.
- Checking the manipulation.
- Obtaining administrative information.

Criteria Affecting Selection of Instruments

- Resources — compensation to data collectors, etc.
- Availability and familiarity.
- Norms and comparability.
- Population appropriateness.
- Administration issues.
- Reputation.

Factors that Contribute to Error of Measurement

- Situational contaminants — participant's awareness.
- Transitory personal factors.
- Response set biases.
- Administration variations.
- Instrument clarity.
- Item sampling.
- Instrument format.

Measure of Quality of Data Collection tool/Instruments:

A. Reliability

Reliability of the tool is defined as consitency with which item is answered accurately.

1. Stability of the instrument is tested by test— retest method.
2. Internal consistency is tested by coefficient alpha for instruments whose items scores are summed.
3. Equivalence through multi-rater kappa and inter-rater kappa.
   - Unreliable instruments reduce statistical power and hence affect statistical conclusion validity of the study.
   - Factors affecting reliability are —
     - Length between two observations,
     - Length of instruments and
     - Heterogeneity of sample.

B. Validity

Validity is defined as the degree to which an instrument measures what it is supposed to measure. There are four types of validity of an instrument. They are —

1. ***Face validity:*** It means the instrument 'looks' as though it is measuring the appropriate construct.
2. ***Content validity:*** Appropriate sample items for measurement of a construct. Representativeness of the questions/items is studied. It is not completely objective as it is based on judgements. Each item should be relevant and accurate. Content Validity Index by expert's evaluation of individual items is calculated.
3. ***Criterion related validity:*** It involves determining the relationship between an instrument and an external criterion called norm/standard established earlier.
   - Said valid when scores correlate highly.
   - Required to have a reliable and valid criterion to compare the instrument.
   - Two types are criterion related validity are:
     - Predictive validity indicating adequacy to differentiate on some future criterion.
     - Concurrent validity indicating ability to distinguish individual items which differ on a present criterion.

4. ***Construct validity:*** It is a key criterion for assessing the quality of study. It concerns inferences from the particulars of the study to the higher order constructs of interest. It measures the abstract of interest. It is:
   a. Vital for development of strong evidence.
   b. Is a challenging task.
   c. Techniques for construct validation are —
      i. Know group techniques
      ii. Hypothesized relationships
      iii. Convergent and discriminant validity, i.e. discriminality
      iv. Factor analysis —confirmatory factor analysis.

C. Sensitivity

It is the ability of a measure to identify a case correctly.

D. Specificity

It is the ability of a measure to identify a non-case correctly.

E. Other indicators

They include the instruments —

- Positive predictive value
- Negative predictive value
- Likelihood ratio
- Efficiency
- Comprehensibility
- Precision
- Speededness
- Range
- Linearity
- Reactivity.

The goal of a data collection plan is to produce data that are of exceptional quality. Every decision the researcher makes about the data collection methods and procedures is likely to affect data quality and hence the resultant findings and quality of evidence. Nurses must judiciously choose their subjects, and sites of data collection, train the data collectors ahead of time and test their skills in pilot study, collect data at appropriate time and maintain the confidentiality of data; to yield good evidence through their studies.

CHAPTER 11 Biostatistics

An investigator is expected to know the application of statistical procedures in order to interpret the findings of his/her study in statistical terms. The interpretations in numerical with statistical confirmations improve the strength of their findings.

DEFINITION

Biostatistics is the science and art of collection, compilation, presentation, analysis and interpretation of numerical data concerned with biological events which are affected by multiple factors.

- It is that branch of statistics where mathematical facts and data are related to biological events like, disease, illness, etc.
- **Vital statistics (Health Statistics):** It is a branch of biostatistics related to vital events in the life such as birth, migration, death, marriages, etc.

Population (Universe): In biostatistics, the term population is used to denote the units under study. It includes all persons, events, objects under study. Population is defined in terms of size, structure, time-frame, geography, and nature.

Sample: Sample is the portion of the population selected by a process called sampling. Instead of studying the entire population only sample is studied.

CHARACTERISTICS OF POPULATION

- It can be finite or infinite in terms of size.
- It can be homogeneous or heterogeneous in terms of composition.
- Population needs to be defined in terms of time or time period.
- Population can be static or dynamic in nature.
- Population can be static for one characteristic but dynamic for another.

Parameter: It is a constant that describes the population.

Statistic: It is a constant that describes the sample.

Attributes: An attribute is a characteristic based on which the population can be divided into categories or classes; e.g., gender, caste, religion, severity grade of a disease, etc.

Variate: It is a characteristic which has a scale of measurement. e.g. height, weight, Hb%, Income, IQ, etc.

A continuous variate is the one which theoretically can assume any value from 0 to infinity. Therefore measurement is in fractions or decimals; e.g., height, weight.

A discrete Variate is the one which even theoretically cannot be measured in fractions or decimals; e.g. size of a family, RBC/WBC count, etc.

Inference: Inference is a process of drawing conclusion based on the data and some statistical applications. The inference can be about magnitude, difference or association, e.g. boys are taller than girls.

Forecasting: Forecasting is a method of making predictions about one characteristic in a unit in population; based on some other characteristic or characteristics. It involves examining the units in population for the characteristics under study and finding out if there exists any pattern in their relationship.

APPLICATIONS OF STATISTICS

A. **Statistics as a numerical data:** Statistics tells us the facts that it deals with figures, counts and measurements. It is thus affected by the collection process and personal bias.

B. **Statistics as a tool:** Statistics provides us with the tools for data collection, presentation, analysis and interpretation.

C. **Statistics as science:** Statistics has a firm foundation of principles, laws, tests and theories. Based on these, the discipline can make firm predictions, due to statistical laws, theory of probability, principle of normal distribution, tests of significance, etc. statistics is a science and hence has wide applications in varied fields like agriculture, weather forecasting, politics and health.

TYPES OF DATA

Data can be classified in following ways:

Based on Characteristic

Qualitative: Relates to attributes,

Quantitative: Quantitative discrete,
Quantitative continuous.

Based on Source

Primary: direct measurement,

Secondary: derived from records, etc.

Based on Field

In computer database management software, data are arranged in tabular form. The columns are called fields and rows are records. Each field can hold record of its type. Common types of fields are character type, numeric type, date type and logical type.

Character type: Name, address, etc.

Numeric type: Age, height, weight, BSL, BP, Sr. No., etc.

Date type: Date of birth, date of admission, date of discharge, etc.
(mm/dd/yyyy) — American format.
(dd/mm/yyyy) — British format.
(yyyy/dd/mm) — ANSI format.

Logical type: This refers to dichotomous data e.g. gender (Male/Female), result of drug trial (cured/not cured), residence (rural/urban), etc.

Based on Contents

Depending on contents, the data can be classified into 4 types:

a. **Nominal data**: Synonym to qualitative data. The data are presented as frequency distribution of some characteristics like gender, religion, etc.
   - The groups do not have any logical order.
   - Names like good/bad, male/female, etc.
   - No implication to adjacent categories.

b. **Ordinal data:** Data is presented according to rank or order.
   - There is logical order but no measurement.
   - No implication of class – interval.
   - The groups are not equidistant.
   - There is no true zero.

c. **Interval data:**
   - Data placed in meaningful intervals and order.
   - There is no implication of ratio.
   - No starting point like zero.
   - Considerable amount of measurement is possible.

d. **Ratio data**: Data are presented in frequency distribution.
   - Logical order.
   - Meaningful groups.
   - Meaningful ratio exists.
   - True zero exists.

Difference in 4 data types

Property	*Nominal data*	*Ordinal data*	*Interval data*	*Ratio data*
Logical order	–	+	+	+
Meaningful Group-interval	–	–	+	+
Meaningful ratio	–	–	–	+
True zero	–	–	–	+

NEED TO IDENTIFY THE TYPE OF DATA

The knowledge of type of data helps us —

1. In further analysis of data.
2. In selection of method for data presentation.
3. In selection of tests for significance.
4. In correct interpretation and forecasting.

COMMON SYMBOLS USED IN STATISTICS

Also called statistical notations

- Σ → Sigma means summation of
- χ^2 → Chi square

- S (σ) → Standard deviation of sample
- μ → (mu) means standard deviation of population
- π → (pie) universal constant obtained by 22/7.
- x → Numeric value of a variable in sample /population
- m → $\bar{x}$ → Arithmetic mean of the variable in given sample.
- M → Arithmetic mean of variable in given population.
- n → Size of sample = no. of observations.
- N → Size of population
- p → Proportion of an attribute in sample.
- P → Proportion of an attribute in population.
- < → Less than
- > → Greater than
- ≠ → Not equal to
- Observations / variable = $x_1, x_2, x_3 \ldots\ldots\ldots x_n$.
- F → Frequency.
- r → Correlation.
- R → No. of rows
- C → No. of columns
- t → Students 't' test
- z → Z test
- f → Analysis
- II → Deviation

SOURCES OF DATA

See Figure 11.1.

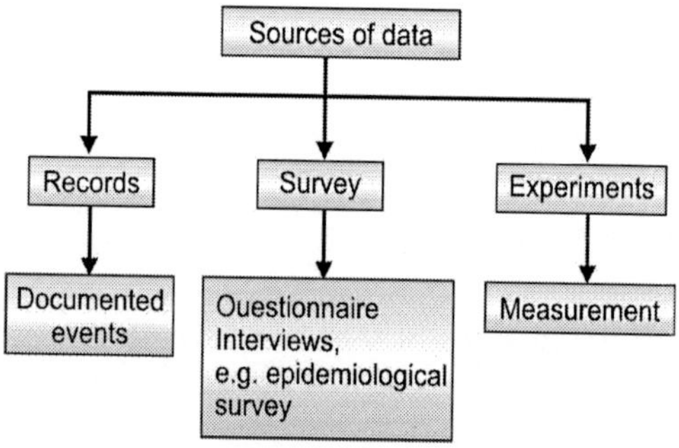

Fig. 11.1: Sources of statistical data

Measurement: The required information is collected by actual measurement in the object, element or person

- Provides primary data, e.g. temperature, BP, etc.

Questionnaire: A standardized and pretested questionnaire in the language of respondents is given and respondents are expected to give the information by answering it.

Success depends on the following:

- Quality of questionnaire.
- The enthusiasm of respondents.
- The ability of respondents to give correct information.
- Useful to collect information about large number of attributes and variates in short-time.

Interview: Used as supplement to questionnaire or independently.

Success depends on the following:

- Rapport established with the respondent.
- Ability of interviewer to extract exact information.
- Readiness of the respondent to share correct information.

Records: Required information may be available in various records like census, survey records, hospital records, service records, etc.

The utility of information depends on the following:

- Uniformity
- Completeness
- Standardization
- Accuracy
- Reasons for which the information was recorded.

PROBLEMS IN DATA COLLECTION

Variation: The term biological variation is used for variation in the measurements in the same individual even if the measurement tool is standardized and the data collector is the same.

Sampling variation is the variation seen in the statistic of two samples drawn from same statistical population.

Mistakes and Errors: They can be of three types —

- Instrumental error/technical error.

- Systematic error.
- Random error.
  - (a) **Instrumental/technical error:** Due to faulty or unstandardized instruments used for data collection.
  - (b) **Systematic error:** Due to a peculiar fault in the machine or technique, e.g. 'zero' of the weighing machine is not adjusted properly. The error repeats in all observations.
  - (c) **Random error:** It is introduced by changes in the conditions in which observations are made or measurements are taken.

PREVENTION OF ERRORS AND MISTAKES

Errors and mistakes can be prevented or minimized by:

- Using standard instruments.
- Using standardized, pretested questionnaire.
- Using trained and skilled persons.
- Using multiple observations and averaging them.
- Using correct recording procedures.
- Applying standard and widely accepted statistical manipulations (calculations)

Bias: It is a systematic error. It results in tendency to produce results that differ in systematic manner from the true values.

Types of bias: There are three main types of bias:

(1) Selection bias (2) Measurement bias (3) Confounding bias.

1. **Selection bias:** When the persons selected for the study systematically differ from those not selected, selection bias occurs.
   - Entry in the study is not random.
   - Selection of volunteers and exclusion of those who do not volunteer or are absent, etc.
2. **Measurement bias:** It is also called classification bias. Faulty instruments result in measurement bias.
3. **Confounding bias:** The dependent and independent variable in a study may be associated with / influenced by a third factor. This is called confounding factor and the bias due to it is called confounding bias. The confounding factor may be -
   - A risk factor for outcome of the study.

- Associated with the cause under study.
- Not a cause of the outcome in the same study.

Measures to overcome the confounding bias —

- Restricting the study to limited number of variables.
- Matching.
- Stratified analysis.
- Multivariate analysis.

PRECAUTIONS IN DATA COLLECTION

Standardization: The comparison is difficult/impossible if data collection methods differ.

- Use of standard pretested questionnaire.
- Use of universally accepted methods and techniques.
- Use of standard definitions for categorization.

All of these help to achieve standardization in a study.

Training: Training of the persons involved in data collection ensures-

- Uniformity
- Accuracy
- Completeness of the data collected.

Training for use of various measurements, use of questionnaire and interview method should be given.

Pretesting: Data collection needs pretesting. It is a sort of mock trial of data collection on a smaller scale.

- Such trial should not include the population in actual study.
- Pretesting helps to avoid:
  - Ambiguities
  - Inaccuracies
  - Uncertainties.
- Provides training for the personnel involved.

Storage: If the time duration between data collection and analysis is expected to be long, the durable storage device for collected data must be used.

- Precomputer age: Registers, folders, cards, punch cards, etc.
- Computer age: added advantage of retrieval— Ease in data presentation and analysis.

- Data must be protected from insects, rats and environmental changes.

COMPILATION OF DATA

Compilation of data involves — (1) Data editing
(2) Data reduction

Data Editing: Data editing is correction for incompleteness, inaccuracies, illegal entries and inconsistencies in data. For example:

- Nonrecording of weight for few students.
- Period of gestation in weeks for few and in months for others.
- Recording age as on 1st Jan for few and for others as on date of data collection.
- An eighteen-year-old mother with 4 children.
- Puerperal sepsis is a cause of death in male.
- Entry of 50 years old woman in the study designed for 15 to 44 years only.

DATA EDITING TECHNIQUES

- Use of standard, pretested formats.
- Detailed instructions with data entry schedule.
- Training of persons involved.
- Supervision.
- Sample checking.
- Checks introduced in data schedule.
- Computerization of data entry.

Data reduction: It is the reduction of voluminous raw data in manageable amount for the purpose of presentation and analysis. Tabulation is the most common method of data reduction. Data reduction involves a compromise between loss of details and compactness achieved.

FREQUENCY DISTRIBUTION

Frequency distribution is the summary of the number of times different values of a variable occur.

- *Simple frequency distribution*: When presented without any data reduction.
- *Grouped frequency distribution:* When presented with data reduction.
- *Relative frequency distribution:* When presented as proportion or percentage of groups.
- *Cumulative frequency distribution:* When presented as total of the previous group/groups frequencies with the present group.

DATA PRESENTATION

Objectives of data presentation:

- To arouse the interest of the readers.
- To achieve data reduction without compromising details.
- To enable readers to have quick grasp and impression.
- To draw meaningful impressions.
- To facilitate further analysis.
- To facilitate communication.

Methods of Data Presentation

- Informal—Text and Semi-tabular.
- Formal—Tables, graphs, centering constants, measures of variation, etc.

Tabular Presentation of Data

Tabular data presentation is most common method of data reduction and involves presentation of raw data in columns and rows.

Precautions in Tabular Presentation

- Table should have a title.
- Title should describe 'what', 'where', and 'when'.
- Title should be clear concise and self explanatory.
- Columns and rows should have appropriate sub titles.

Types of Tables

Reference table or master table: This table shows all variables. It contains all the result of data reduction.

Correlation table: This shows two quantitative variables cross classified in many classes. It is used to calculate correlation coefficient (r), e.g. See Table 11.1.

Table 11.1: Height in cms and weight in kg of 440 college students

Weight in kg	*Height in cms 150-154.9*	*Height in cms 155-159.9*	*Height in cms 160-164.9*	*Height in cms 165-169.5*
40-44.9	50	10	10	10
45-49.9	30	50	20	20
50-54.9	20	30	50	30
55-59.9	10	20	20	50

Association table: This table shows association between two qualitative variables. It is also required for calculating sensitivity and specificity of screening test, e.g. see Table 11.2.

Table 11.2: Association between amniocentesis and Ultrasonography test

Amniocentesis	*Ultrasonography*		
	Positive	*Negative*	*Total*
Positive	100	10	110
Negative	05	85	90
Total	105	95	200

Two by two frequency table: This table just shows frequency distribution of two variables or two classes, e.g. see Table 11.3.

Table 11.3: Gender distribution of students in two colleges

College	*Male*	*Female*	*Total*
Medical	600	400	1000
Engineering	500	500	1000
Total	1100	900	2000

Text table: It is a descriptive table. It does not contain any numerical data, e.g. see Table 11.4

Table 11.4: Some information about the siblings

Name	*Residence*	*Occupation*
VD Tendolkar	Belgaum	Lecturer
BK Kulkarni	Nagpur	Lecturer
SK Diwe	Amraovati	Tax consultant

Contingency/complex table: This table contains complex data of two or more variables. It also gives the relationship between two or more variables, e.g. see table 11.5

Table 11.5: Thriving of preterm babies (400) with combination of stimuli

Time	*Tactile stimulus*		*Auditory stimulus*	
	M	*F*	*M*	*F*
15 min	201	199	256	144
30 min	140	260	150	250
45 min	180	220	152	248

Graphical Presentation of Data

Graphical presentation is a visual presentation of data.

Its features are as follows:

- It makes data interesting.
- It makes data easy to understand even to illiterate persons.
- Gives meaningful impression even before the actual analysis of data.

Precautions in Pictorial Presentation

- Each graph should have a self explanatory title.
- The scales for both the axis (x and y) should start from zero.
- The scale should be indicated, with unit of measurement at an appropriate place in the presentation.
- Break in the continuity should be shown with a broken line.
- Key should be self explanatory.

Types of Graph

1. Bar graph.
2. Histogram.
3. Pictogram.
4. Pie diagram.
5. Line diagram.
6. Scatter diagram.
7. Proportionate bar graph.
8. Proportionate line diagram.

Bar Graph or Bar Chart or Bar Diagram

This type of graph is indicated for qualitative and quantitative discrete data.

- Variables are depicted as bars of equal breadth.
- Length of the bar is proportional to the frequency of variables.
- Distance between the bars is equal to or ½ the breadth of the bars.
- The bars may be horizontal or vertical.
- In simple bar chart a single variable is depicted.
- A multiple bar chart, (MBC) exhibits more than one variable.
- Maximum number of variables depicted in a single bar chart is four (Figs 11.2 and 11.3).

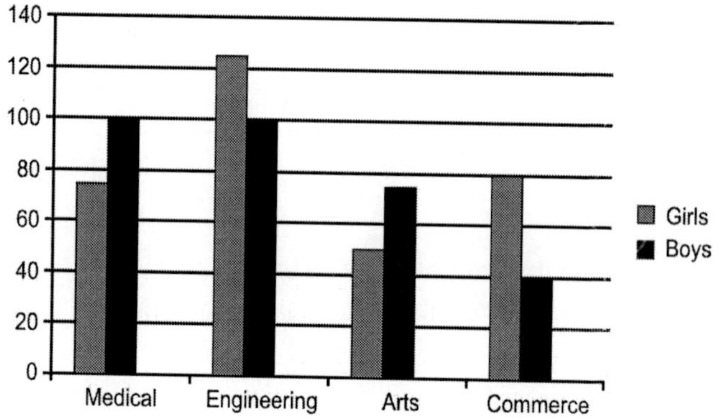

Fig 11.2 : Gender-wise strength of students in different faculties at wardha

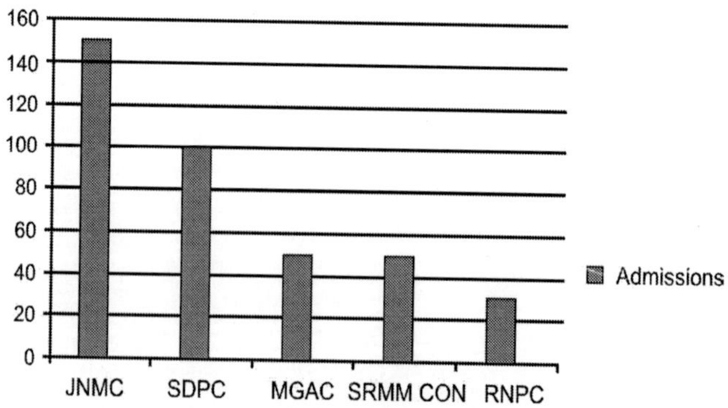

Fig. 11.3: Admission capacity of DMIMS for UG health science courses

Proportionate Bar Chart

In this bar chart, instead of absolute frequency, a proportion (or percentage) of variables is depicted (Fig. 11.4).

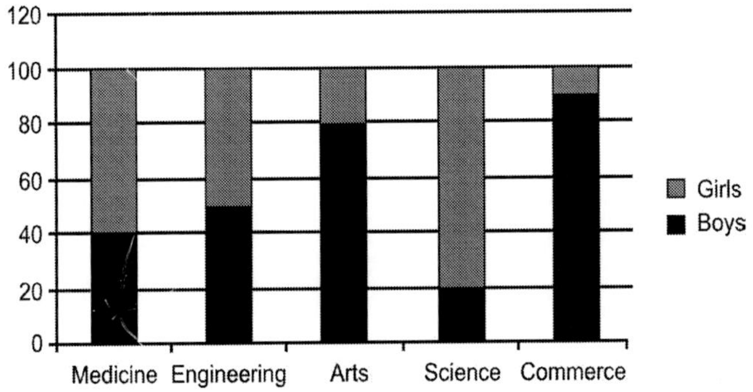

Fig. 11.4: Proportionate bar chart: Proportional distribution of boys and girls in different courses

Pie Diagram or Pie Chart

This type of presentation is indicated for qualitative and quantitative discrete type of data. The frequency of a variable is compared as a segment of a circle (Fig. 11.5).

Segment allocation to frequency of variable A is given by the formula

Seg of A = A × $\frac{360}{N}$ where N is the number in sample size (total observations)

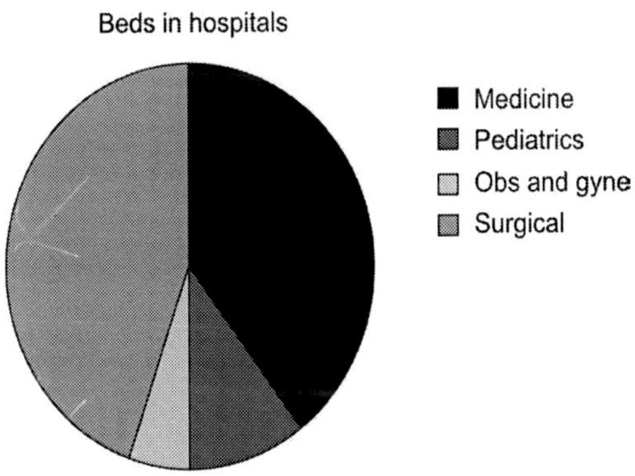

Fig. 11.5 : Distribution of beds in a hospital

Histogram

Histogram is a method of choice for quantitative continuous data.

It is an area diagram consisting of series of adjacent blocks.

Entire area covered by the rectangles denotes total frequency.

The area covered by the individual block represents the variable frequency for that block.

Histogram can deal with unequal class interval data (Fig. 11.6).

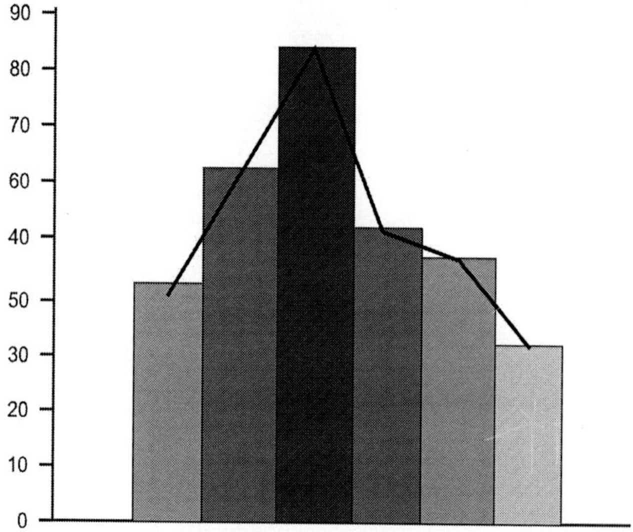

Fig. 11.6 : Histogram and frequency polygon

Frequency Polygon

It is a linear representation of histogram. The centers of top of each rectangle are joined by a line.

Histogram and frequency polygon are difficult to understand. Hence, they are not very popular.

Line Diagram

Line diagram is used to represent change in frequency of a characteristic over a period of time.

- This can uncover trend, if any.

- The change is presumed to be continuous and hence, one can forecast or predict the frequency of the variable at anytime outside the range of observation is called extrapolation.
- Estimating the frequency of variable at anytime within the range of observation is called interpolation.

Proportionate Line Diagram

When the frequency of variable at one of the extreme period is presumed to be 1 or 100 and frequency of other periods is computed proportionately and line diagram is drawn, it is called proportionate line diagram (Figs 11.7 and 11.8).

- Used to compare the proportionate change in two variables over a period of time.

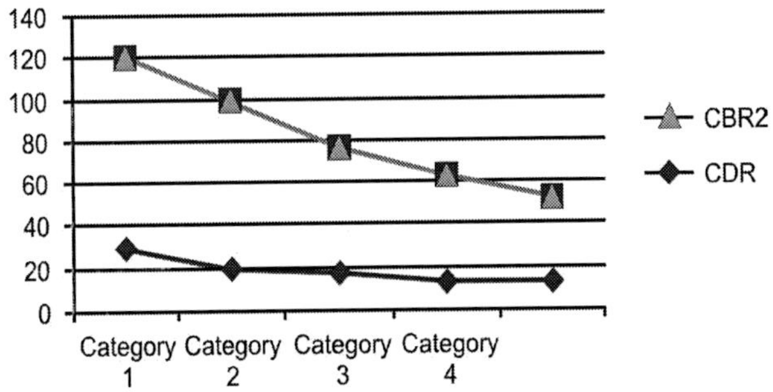

Fig. 11.7: CDR and CBR in India 1941-1991

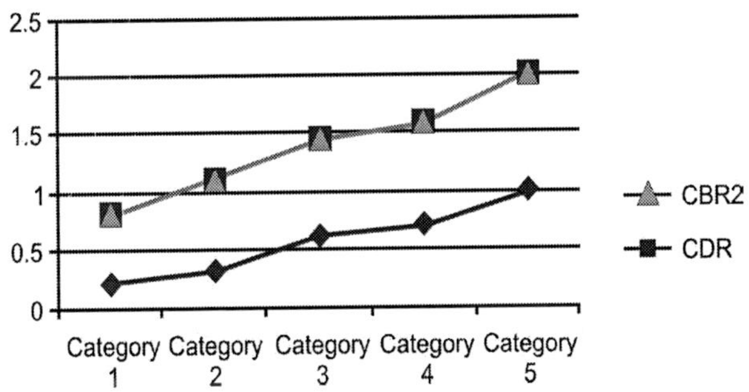

Fig. 11.8: CDR and CBR: India 1941-1991 Relative decline

Scatter Diagram

This graphical presentation is used to show relationship, if any, between two quantitative variables.

- X – axis → independent variable.
- Y – axis → dependent variable.
- The general direction (trend) of the dots on graph indicates, whether there is any positive or negative correlation in the two variables.
- The line of containing maximum points is called line of correlation (regression) (Fig. 11.9).

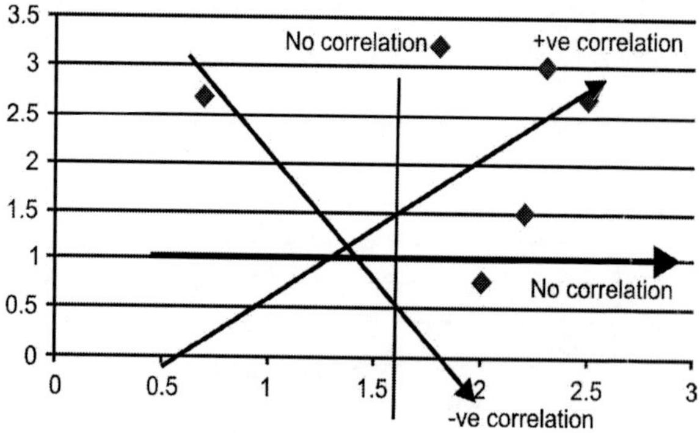

Fig. 11.9: Scatter diagram

Pictogram

This method is indicated for qualitative or quantitative discrete data.

Frequency of a variable is displayed alongside a picture which has some resemblance to the characteristic depicted (Fig. 11.10)

For Example: – Human population
– Population of trees

In pictogram the frequency of each picture should be given.

For Example – 500 human population
– 250 tree population

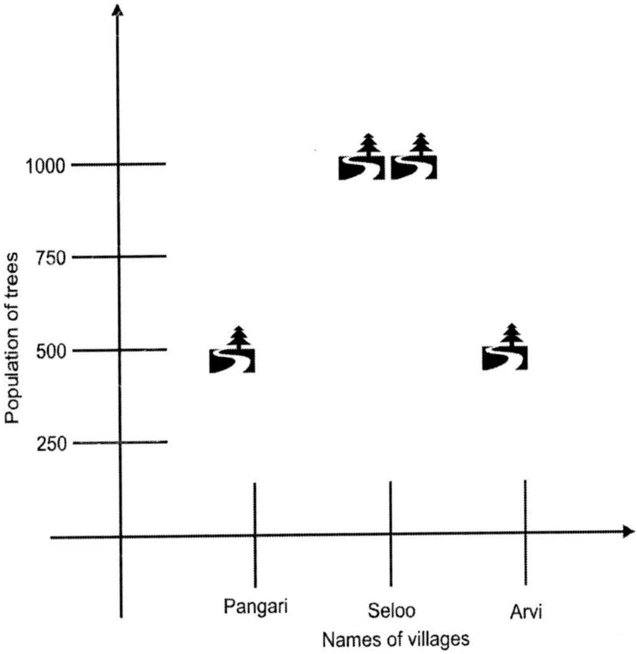

Fig. 11.10: Pictogram of population of trees in selected villages

Spot Map

Spot map is used to show occurrences of events with reference to geographic locations (Fig. 11.11).

Useful tool for showing 'place distribution' in epidemiological studies.

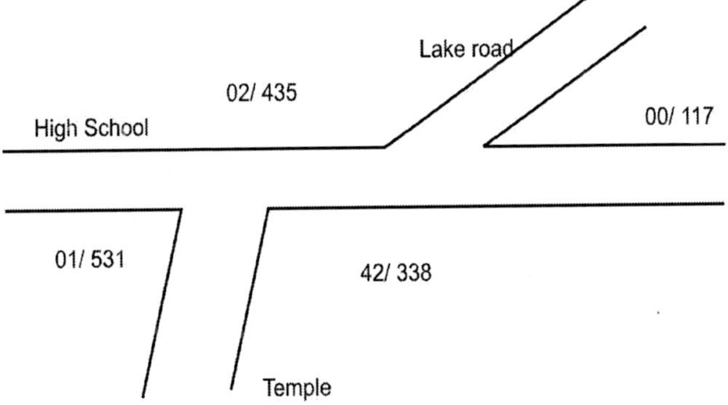

Fig. 11.11: Spot Map: Typhoid cases in a village

Inference: It is clear from this map that there is some problem (typhoid cases are more) in the south east sector of the village that needs investigation.

Epidemic Curve

Epidemic curve is used to show the occurrences of events with passage of time. It is used to present "Time distribution" in epidemiological studies (Fig. 11.12).

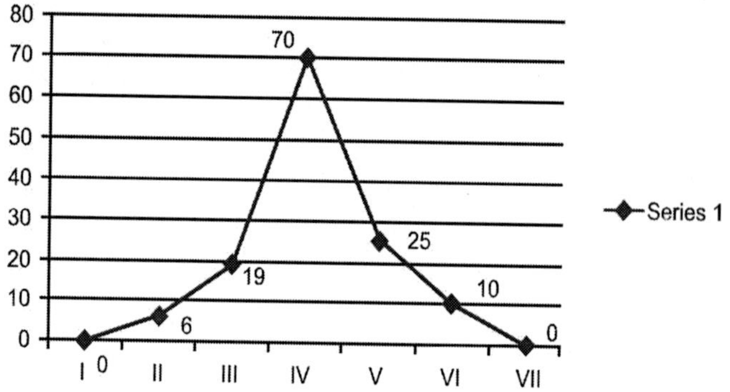

Fig. 11.12 : Weekly distribution of cholera in an outbreak

MEASURES OF CENTRAL TENDENCY

Synonym - Centering constants, measures of averages

Three types of centering constants are used:

- Mean
- Mode
- Median

MERITS OF CENTERING CONSTANTS

- They are easy to calculate.
- They are easy to understand.
- They are rigidly defined.
- They are based on all observations.
- They have sampling stability.

Mean

It is the summation of all observations divided by total number of observations

$$x = mean = \frac{\Sigma_{i=1}^{n} x_i}{n}$$

When only 'n' number of observations are given.

1. *Arithmetic mean:* Arithmetic mean is affected by all the observations as each contributes to its calculation.

   Effects of extreme values is more than that of nearer to mean ones.

2. When frequencies of observations are given then mean is calculated by summation of product of frequency and observation divided by total number of frequencies.

   If $x_1, x_2, \ldots, x_n$ are observations with $f_1, f_2, \ldots, f_n$ as respective frequencies.

$$\therefore \quad x = \frac{x_1 f_1 + x_2 f_2 + \ldots + x_n f_n}{f_1 + f_2 + \ldots + f_n}$$

$$= \frac{\Sigma_{i=1}^{n} x_i f_i}{\Sigma_{i=1}^{n} f_i} = \frac{\Sigma_{i=1}^{n} x_i f_i}{N}$$

3. When means of two different groups of observations is given then combined mean is calculated as—

$$x_n = \frac{n_1 x_1 + n_2 x_2}{n_1 + n_2}$$

   Therefore, in general

$$x_n = \frac{n_1 x_1 + n_2 x_2 + \ldots + n_n x_n}{n_1 + n_2 + \ldots + n_n}$$

$$x_n = \frac{\Sigma_{i=1}^{n} n_i x_i}{\Sigma_{i=1}^{n} n_i}$$

4. *Weighted mean*: When weights of the observation are given

   Observations: $x_1, x_2, \ldots, x_n$

   Weights: $w_1, w_2, \ldots, w_n$

$$x_w = \frac{\Sigma_{i=1}^{n} x_i w_i}{\Sigma_{i=1}^{n} n_i}$$

5. *Geometric mean* → calculated by the formula,
   G = Geometric mean = n^{th} root of product of 'n' number of observations
   $= (x_1, x_2, \ldots, x_n)^{1/n}$

$$\log G = \frac{1}{n}\log\left(x_1 \times x_2 \times \ldots . \times x_n\right)$$

$$\log G = \frac{1}{n}\left(\log x_1 + \log x_2 + \ldots . + \log x_n\right)$$

$$\log G = \frac{1}{n}\left[\sum_{i=1}^{n} \log x_i\right]$$

$$anti\log(\log G) = G = anti\log\left[\frac{1}{n}\sum_{i=1}^{n} \log x_i\right]$$

6. *Harmonic mean:* It is reciprocal of arithmetic mean to the reciprocal of total number of observations.
   H = Harmonic mean

$$= \frac{1}{\frac{1}{n}\Sigma_{i=1}^{n}\frac{1}{x_i}}$$

$$= \frac{\frac{1}{\Sigma_{i=1}^{n}\frac{1}{x_i}}}{n}$$

$$= \frac{n}{\Sigma_{i=1}^{n}\frac{1}{x_i}}$$

Median

It is also called as positional mean. It is the middle observation if the observations in a given series, are arranged in ascending or descending order.

When the number of observations is an even number then the mean of two middle observation is termed as median, e.g.

Even	*odd*
2	10
3	15
5	17
7	

$$median = \frac{3+5}{2} = 4$$

Mode

It is the most frequently occurring observation. It is the observation that has maximum frequency in a given sample. Sometimes, mode is ill defined. When two or more observations have highest frequency, the sample is called multimodal sample.

Relation between Mean, Median and Mode

The formula for relation between mean, median and mode is given by Karl Pearson.

Mean – Mode = 3 (Mean – Median)

Mean < Median < Mode

In a graphical presentation, mode lies between mean and median.

Normally the curve is symmetrical (Fig. 11.13)

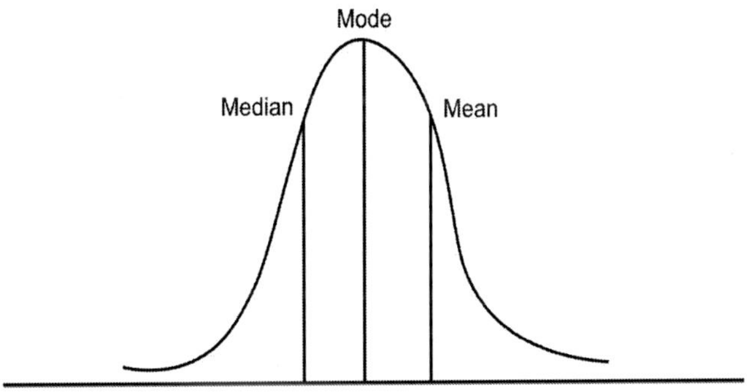

Fig. 11.13: Relationship between mean, median, and mode

COLLECTION OF DEMOGRAPHIC DATA

The different sources for collection of demographic data are:

- Population census
- Records of vital statistics
- Records of health departments
- Records of health institutions
- Reports of special surveys
- Periodic publications by:
  i. Word Health Organization (WHO)
  ii. Registrar General, India.
  iii. Directorate General Health Services (DGHS), New Delhi.
  iv. State Health Directorates.
- Miscellaneous including other health agencies and medical establishments like hospital and nursing homes.

POPULATION CENSUS

Population census is an important source of health information. Census is carried out to assess the national needs and plan programs for the people's welfare. Characteristic features of the census are:

- Full count of population which includes each and every individual and is carried out at regular intervals. First census was conducted in the year 1872 and the next in 1881. Since then, it is being done every ten years and the last one was conducted in 2001. Data collection of 2011 census is in progress at present.
- It pertains to a particular territory and the information is collected by making house to house visit on the specified dates in the first quarter of the first year of each decade.

The census in India is conducted under the Indian Census Act, 1948. Government is responsible for appointing a Census Commissioner. The Registrar General of India is assigned an ex-officio charge of Census Commissioner. The overall census plan is prepared in conformity with 'Principles and Recommendations for National Population Census, United Nations'. Educate people on the importance of census. Preparation of census schedules their pretesting, pilot study and training of enumerators.

Topics covered are as under:

- Total population at the time of census.
- Age, gender, composition and marital status.
- Languages spoken, education and economic status.
- Fertility, i.e. number of children born alive between two censuses to all women up to the date of census.
- Citizenship, place of birth, urban and rural populations.

Uses of a Population Census in Health Matters

- The census determines population of area which forms basis for calculation of health indices such as birth, fertility, death, morbidity, marriage rates, etc.
- All health services are planned and community measures are adopted as per nature and size of the population.
- Average rate of growth of population per year is computed from the population enumerated in two census years.
- Knowledge of population distribution helps in planning of the other welfare services such as provision of schools, orphanages, food supplies, etc.

LIFE TABLE

Life table is a special type of cohort analysis which takes into account the life history of a hypothetical group or cohort of people that decreases gradually by death till all members of the group died.

USES AND APPLICATION

- To find the number of survivors at birth or at any age.
  - At the age of 5, to find the number of children likely to enter primary school.
  - At the age of 15, to find the number of women entering fertile period or find the number of adolescents entering the community.
  - At the age of 18, to find the number of persons who become eligible for voting : at 55 or 58 or 60, who become eligible for pension; and at 65 and over, to assess the geriatric problems and solutions like income tax benefits, railway concession, etc.

  - At the age of 45 or above, to find the number of women reaching menopause.
  - Survival at different ages of women in fertile period and birth of female children from the age birth to 15 years, which helps in finding age-wise fertility rate, net reproduction rate, etc.
- To estimate the number likely to die after joining service till retirement, helping, thereby in budgeting for payment towards risk or pension.
- To find expectation of life or longevity of life at birth or any other age.
- To find survival rate after treatment in a chronic disease like diabetes and hypertension by modified life table technique.

In short, life table helps to project population estimates by age and gender. It is also called as biometer of population. To construct a life table, two things are required:

- Population living at all individual ages in a selected year.
- Number of deaths that occurred in these ages during the selected year.

Thus vital statistics means data which gives quantitative information on vital events occurring in life, i.e. migration, births, marriages, and deaths in a given population. They form essential tools in any demographic study. The studies conducted in health sector use demographic data to a considerable extent.

CHAPTER

12 Computers in Research

The science and technology is embracing new heights every day. This has great impact on the health care delivery system. Computer technology and internet facilities have reduced the world into global village. It has immensely helped the researchers to manage voluminous data of their study into small chips that can be carried in pockets. Naturally the enthusiasm of researchers is multiplied as they are spared of tedious calculations and manual handling of bulky data which used to restrict their field of study.

COMPUTER REVOLUTION

Twenty first century is predominantly ruled by computers. In the development process, the size of a computer has shrunk and the power has increased.

Application of computers in health sector can be studied as under:

- Methods in biostatistics
- Community or public health care.
- Hospital establishments, nursing homes and clinics of academic general practitioners.
- Health sciences research.

Application in Biostatistics

Computers are used for—

- Collection, compilation, tabulation and diagrammatic presentation in the manner required for any size of data for completeness and accuracy.
- Finding averages: coefficient of variation, standard deviation and standard error and percentiles, etc. of any size of data simultaneously.
- The application of tests of significance such as 'Z', 't' and χ^2 correlation and regression coefficients and other tests to find probability (p values), necessary in practice of medicine, public health and in research.

- Construction of life tables.
- Probability of length of life in any chronic disease, e.g. cancer without or after operation.
- Chances of survival and period of survival.

Application in Community or Public Health Care and Management

To formulate policy, monitor implementation and finally to evaluate it, the prime need data. Computer based 'Health information' systems have been described as a necessity by WHO.

Computers have great capacity for storage of past and present data which helps in comparison of events in the past. A very familiar example is prevalence rate of tuberculosis which in 1958 and today in 1997 is same in spite of specific and effective drugs at our command and reduction in period of treatment from 3 years to 8 months allowing mobility and gradually normal work during treatment also.

Forecasting of epidemics: Computers can help in that more precisely and effectively. That helps in modification of measures in prevention and control.

Application of Computers in Hospital Establishments

- Increase efficiency and improve services to the patients for better professional care in computerized methods of diagnosis using cat scan angiography, biopsy before surgery and computer aided treatment as by laser in stone crushing in urinary system and electrical vaporization in enlargement of prostate.
- Prevent losses due to errors and pilferage and reduce overheads and salaries and tighter management of control to enhance image of establishment.
- Computerize full range of drug reference systems by keeping check over stocks of drugs and their expiry date and standard recommendation of doses of different drugs.
- Save time over non-clinical work like quick retrieval of records, spending less time on each revisit of the patient and quicker billing, etc.

- Scheduling of appointments to reduce waiting periods for the patients, manage routine documents such as growth charts, follow-up of patients including progress, visits, immunization, etc.
- Keeping academic references – statistics and reference material for preparation and presentation of papers and slides, thus keeping communications with others around the world.

Computers are used in the areas where humans are deficient like in fast calculations, storage and retrieving a large amount of information, searching for specific information and drawing for geographical distribution, colour manipulation, etc. Thus these are the areas where computers can help immensely.

Computers are very versatile in the areas such as patients' records, reports of investigations, inventory, billing and accounts.

Computerized medical records are very efficient, quick to locate, accurate space saving and long lasting. Computerized sheets are complete, systematic, consistent, legible, quick, less cost-wise and give a lot of information.

Inventory: It is extremely difficult to maintain inventory details manually especially with several thousand items like drugs, instruments, linen and furniture, etc. in the hospital. Computerized systems are helpful in checking billing and accounts. Obviated long queues, totaling mistakes, wrong entries and quarrelling of patients are the hallmarks of manual accounts.

Diagnosis: Computers can be used as an aid to assist practitioners to prescribe right medicine. Lots of information in terms of formulations available, symptoms, case histories, etc. can be stored and accessed by one press of a key. If the doctor himself is free he can make a probable diagnosis and give provisional treatment on the basis of probabilities. Today, devices are available which can be connected to central computer at the medical center remotely over telephone lines from a patient's home.

COMPUTERS IN RESEARCH

Researchers in health care need to analyze data to understand and report significant observation for which large value of data must be analyzed. Computers make this possible and in a short time.

Programs to support statistical analysis have made the task easier. Some of the statistical packages widely used are —

EXCEL, LOTUS 123, MULTIPLAN, DBASE3+, HELIX, OMNIS, Rbase, REFLEX, BMDP, SAS-PC, SPSS-PC, SYSTAT, Minitab, Genstat, GLIM, EPI-INFO.

The computers still have not solved one problem, the right analysis for the data available, i.e. Statistical Expert System to select the appropriate statistical analysis for the available data. The computer is not 'brain' and 'smart'. It is simply an obdient servant.

INTERNET

It is an information express highway. It signifies a global network of computers that are linked by satellite, telephone, etc. Internet helps to review the literature worldwide, keeps us informed about the latest status of research projects in different parts of the world. In addition, it aids in fast dissemination of results of study projects so that multisite studies can be conducted promptly to enhance the strength of the evidence in a study. Internet also provides for real discussion with experts for efficient guidance.

This means computers are at our call round a clock. One does not even step out of the house to get the required information. It is just a 'click' away. No wonder the world is shrinking and knowledge platforms are expanding.

Bibliography

1. Nursing Research: Generating and Assessing Evidence for Nursing Practice — Denise E Polit and Cheryl Tatano Beck.
2. Foundations of Nursing — Potter and Perry.
3. Nursing Now! — Joseph T Catalano.
4. Nursing Research— BT Basavanthappa.
5. Principles And Practice of Biostatistics — Dr JV Dixit.
6. Leddy and Pepper's Conceptual Bases of Professional Nursing — Hood Lucy and Susan Kun Leddy.
7. Nursing in Today's World — Ellis Janice and Celia Love Hartley.
8. Research Methodology: Method and Techniques — CR Kothari.
9. Psychiatric Mental Health Nursing Research Digest— Joyce J Fitpatrick and Patricia A Wike.

Index